In *Children's Food: The Good, the Bad and the Useless*, Dr Lobstein unravels the mysteries whose interests official regulations [...] ing. He demonstrates how [...] manufacturers and distrib[...] [...] se of the consumer. He highlights p[...] [...]ks and dangers that we run when we buy fo[...] our children and he decodes the mysteries of food labels.

Dr Lobstein ends on a practical note by describing what a properly balanced diet should contain, and he lists the types of food that really are good for children.

Dr Lobstein is the specialist on children's food and nutrition at the London Food Commission, Britain's independent food watchdog, whose book, *Food Adulteration and How to Beat It* was published by Unwin Hyman in July 1988.

CHILDREN'S FOOD

The good, the bad and the useless

Tim Lobstein PhD

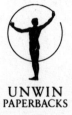

UNWIN
PAPERBACKS

LONDON SYDNEY WELLINGTON

First published in paperback by Unwin®Paperbacks, an imprint of Unwin Hyman Limited in 1988.

UNWIN HYMAN LIMITED
15/17 Broadwick Street
London W1V 1FP

Allen & Unwin Australia Pty Ltd
8 Napier Street, North Sydney, NSW 2060, Australia

Allen & Unwin New Zealand Pty Ltd with Port Nicholson Press
60 Cambridge Terrace, Wellington, New Zealand

British Library Cataloguing in Publication Data

Lobstein, Tim
    Children's food.
1. Processed food. Nutritional values.
I. Title.
641.1
ISBN 0–04–440300–3

Typeset in Garamond Original 10 on 11 point
by Computape (Pickering) Ltd, Pickering, North Yorkshire
and printed in Great Britain by
Cox and Wyman Ltd, Reading.

Contents

Preface

Young children represent a huge market for the makers of processed food. Even before school age, children in Britain are consuming an estimated 50 million meals each week, worth over a billion pounds annually to the food industry. And even before their first birthday, children are starting down the path towards the record quantities of sweets and crisps, biscuits, soft drinks and ice creams consumed in Britain, a market worth over 8 billion pounds annually.

The quantity and nature of manufactured food now being eaten have never been known before. Never have we been offered so many different products, using such a range of processing techniques. Never have children been exposed to such a diet of manufactured, refined and processed foods, in such a range and variety, so expertly sold to catch the eyes and the minds of small girls and boys. From the very first weeks of life, little children and their anxious parents are a 'target market' for food companies keen to promote their products.

Is this a good or bad thing? Are children now able to get a far better diet than before, or have things gone downhill? Young children are most in need of a nutritious diet, with adequate minerals and vitamins for their growing bodies, to set them up for a lifetime of good health. Is this what they are getting? Is nutritious food cheaper than ever or are we being overwhelmed by junk?

This book looks at the bewildering array of foods available for children from their earliest days and offer ways of judging what is good and what is bad – and what may be downright useless – on the shelves of our shops today. It also considers the current dietary recommendations being made by professional health workers and how these can best be met from the foods available to us. It gives tables showing the nutrients children need to grow healthily, and the foods that can give these nutrients. And it considers the strategies and tactics in a parent's continuing battle to keep their children healthy.

Being responsible for growing children is a difficult enough task without having to fight off the food companies and their inappropriate products. The manufacturers spend millions of pounds every day promoting their wares and developing new combinations of ingredients and additives. Only occasionally can a few small voices of dissent and criticism get heard. This book is one of them.

We feel that the promotion that food manufacturers give to themselves and to their products needs to be balanced by the voice of the consumer. Consumers don't have millions of pounds to spend and rarely get to speak out. Because of the lack of balance, this book will only occasionally congratulate manufacturers for their good practices. After all, they congratulate themselves often enough, and we don't need to add to that. Consumers should *expect* good practices, and speak out against bad ones: so we make no apology for focusing on the problems, the bad practices and the shortfalls of the food industry, and leave them to advertise their good points as they do every day.

Acknowledgements

Much of the material in this book actually comes from the work of people other than myself. In particular I owe whole paragraphs, and much inspiration, to Chris Griffin and Dave Thomas of Wigan Social Services, Helen Strange of Southwark Social Services, Shirley Gunder Forbes of Islington Social Services and Julie Sheppard of the London Food Commission.

I also want to thank the staff of the London Food Commission and the many people who read drafts of this book and supported me during its creation, in particular the following individuals:

Issy Cole-Hamilton and Tim Lang
Kathy Adams
Rosemary Davies
Sinead Fleming
Dr Sue Hunt
Ros Lowe
Gay Palmer and Patti Rundall
Aubrey Sheiham
Gill Shinkwin
Lyn Stockley

who bear no responsibility for the final product, except that it would not have come into existence without them.

This book has been inspired by the work of Caroline Walker.

PROLOGUE

Stop, reader, stop; shed not a tear —
The food trade is not buried here
But nor's it praised.
                          Your feelings hold
For us to whom the food is sold
Who cannot boast in magazines
Or puff ourselves on TV screens
But have to trust that what we buy
Is genuinely nutritious and
        delicious and economical and
            wholesome and fun for
                our children to try!

1   Trouble in Store

WE NEED FOOD

It might be technically possible to put all our food needs into one capsule, to be taken when we get up and then we eat nothing for the rest of the day.

But until that day comes we all have to eat. *What* we eat is obviously important. What children eat is particularly important: they are still growing and they are more vulnerable to infections, pollutants and other drains on their physical resources.

Food provides the raw materials for growth and for defence against illness, injury and poisons in the environment. Specifically it provides:

energy   measured in calories
protein   essential for all the body's cells
fats   to be burnt for energy, and some types of fat – *essential
    fatty acids* – for artery, nerve and brain growth
dietary fibre   for a healthy digestive system
vitamins   the essential chemicals we need but cannot make
    ourselves
minerals   some of which are also essential in our diet
water   to replace what we lose (and we lose water with every
    breath we take)

Food comes in great variety. Roots, berries, leaves, seeds, eggs, birds, insects, fish, meat, animal milk and mothers' milk – the human diet is an endless pattern of different combinations of materials found in nature, which can provide the nourishment we need. That is the *theory*, but with the development of sophisti- cated agricultural methods, highly technical processing operations and complex long-storage techniques for warehouse and retail shelves, the *practice* is now very different from what has gone before. Many of our foods nowadays would be largely unrecognisable to our ancestors, even of only a century ago. The last few decades alone have seen a huge rise in the amount of processed foods we buy – estimated now to account for 80 per cent or more of what we spend on food.

Now, with a new interest in healthy eating, parents are getting anxious that they may not be giving the right food to their children, and that left to themselves children will just choose the junk and rubbish which parents are most unhappy about. Manufacturers have started putting labels on their foods saying how good each one is – 'no added this', 'enriched with that', 'your complete daily vitamins in one portion' and so on.

But is this healthy food? What do children need and what are they actually getting? If they are not getting everything they need, or are getting too much of something they don't need, then will this do them any harm? And who benefits from this?

IT'S ALL VERY STRANGE

'This junk food – I mean – it can't be really bad for you or it wouldn't be allowed, would it?'

The trouble is, as we shall see in this book, that the present food regulations *do* allow all manner of odd labelling practices and strange food processing techniques that raise serious questions about the possible damage to our children's health. Many of the products we buy in the food stores today have never been eaten before. Young, growing children may be particularly vulnerable to these unusual, inappropriate foods and untested chemicals. They could be heading into a whole lot of trouble.

Compare these labels from a baby's first foods (Figs. 1–3). This one looks healthy.

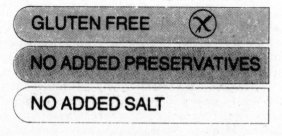

Figure 1.1

This one seems even better. Look at the long list.

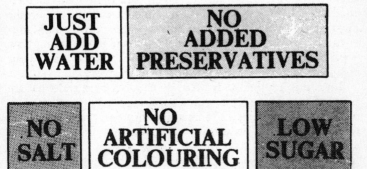

Figure 1.2

But what about this – it's remembered about egg and milk.

GLUTEN FREE

NO ADDED SALT

EGG FREE

MILK FREE

NO ADDED PRESERVATIVES

**NO ARTIFICIAL COLOURS
OR FLAVOURS**

Figure 1.3

CONFUSED?

And what about a baby's first drinks? There's been a lot of fuss about sugar in the rose-hip syrup. So now every manufacturer tries to convince you that their product has hardly any at all (Fig. 1.4)!

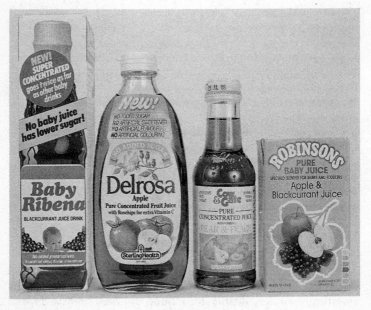

Figure 1.4

The first ingredient in Baby Ribena is a form of sugar (glucose syrup). But they claim that it is still better than those that don't add sugar.
PUZZLED?

For twenty years we have known that some food additives – such as the bright food colourings that children find attractive – can provoke asthma, skin rashes and behavioural problems in susceptible children. Several additives are in fact banned from foods if the foods are marketed for babies and young children.

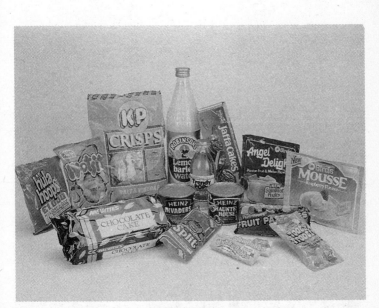

Figure 1.5

All these foods (Fig. 1.5) contain the banned additives – so if the manufacturers were ever to claim that these foods were designed specifically to be suitable for young children they could be breaking the law. (NB. These products were all purchased in 1987 or 1988. However, manufacturers are changing their ingredients (perhaps under pressure from publicity like this!) so it is possible that for some products the banned additives will have been removed by the time you read this book.)

ALARMED?

These 'Low-Sugar' rusks (Fig. 1.6) for teething babies to chew on seem a good idea. But the sugar content is higher than doughnuts or currant buns!

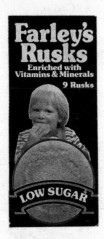 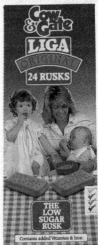

Figure 1.6

Drinks such as these (Fig. 1.7) can have more added sugars than Coca-Cola. They may be called 'Whole Orange' drinks, but they are *not* wholly made of oranges. They are made of the whole of an orange – flesh, pith and skin – plus added sugar and water.

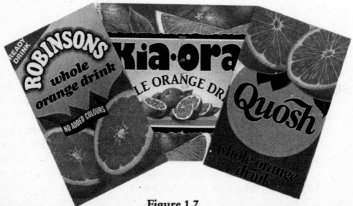

Figure 1.7

And the 'all natural' additives used to make these sweets attractive include chemicals derived from crushed cactus-beetles and their eggs, burnt vegetables and flamingo feathers (Fig. 1.8).

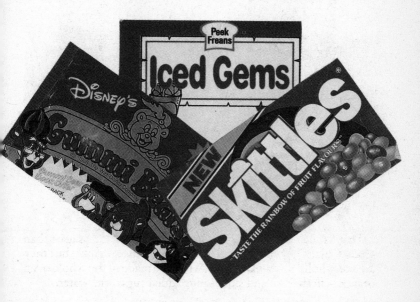

Figure 1.8

SUSPICIOUS?

Apart from the Vitamin C, this drink provides sugar and water and very little else nutritionally (Fig. 1.9). It has stopped calling itself a health drink.

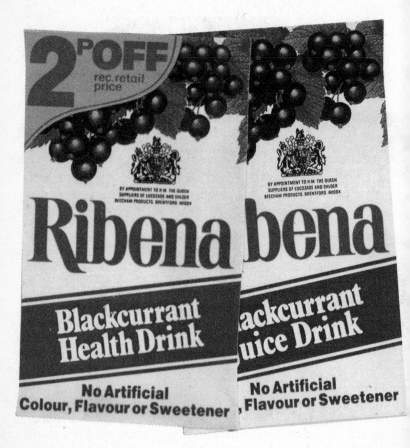

Figure 1.9

But these similar products (Fig. 1.10) still claim to be health drinks, or to imply that they play a useful role in a healthy diet.

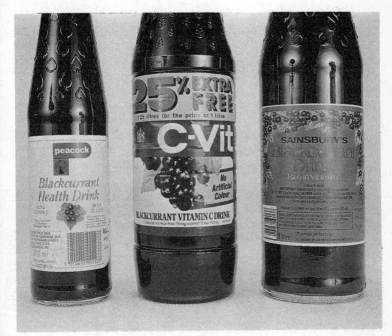

Figure 1.10

Both the second and third of these contain saccharin (a chemical not permitted in food marketed for babies or young children) and several other chemicals (benzoates, sulphites and azo dyes) associated with ill health in some children. Yet the second bottle recommends giving the drink to children from one year of age, and the third describes how to dilute the drink for 'babies and young children'.

SHOCKED?

The government's advisory committee on infant nutrition has recommended mothers not to add salt to an infant's diet, and they call on manufacturers to exercise caution in the addition of salt to infant food products.

Here are two pamphlets for mothers (Figs. 1.11, 1.12) The first one says 'don't add salt to the food your baby eats'.

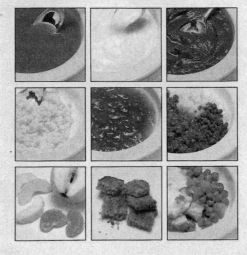

Figure 1.11

The second one says you can give your 6-month-old baby 'the good savoury taste of Marmite' on toast. Marmite is about 10 per cent pure salt.

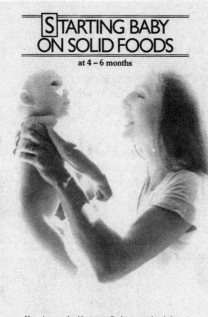

Figure 1.12

The first came from the Health Education Council (now the Health Education Authority), a non-commercial body funded by the government. The second is produced by Marmite Ltd and is sent in quantities to NHS children's clinics by company staff. PERPLEXED?

A WHOLE NEW WORLD OF EATING

Are we right to feel confused, puzzled, alarmed, suspicious, shocked or perplexed? Is what we eat, and what our children eat, very different from, say, ten, twenty or thirty years ago? And was it better for us then, or is it better now?

As a nation we have taken to eating processed foods more than virtually any other country in the world. This isn't necessarily something to be worried about – there are processes and processes. For many vegetables the freezing process does little harm, and as the vegetables are likely to be frozen the day they are picked, and eaten the day they are thawed, they may well be better quality than if they had stood around in warehouses and on the greengrocer's shelf for up to a week or more.

But the supermarket freezer today contains much more than frozen vegetables. Now we are offered frozen pies, burgers, ready-to-serve meals – everything from fish and chips to ice cream. And although by no means everyone has a freezer, the overall trend is large enough to show on the national statistics of what households are eating.

Take frozen meat products – which includes frozen burgers, pies, sausage rolls, frozen cooked meats and ready meals – compared with the nation's favourite fresh meat, beef (Table 1.1).

Table 1.1
(amount per person per year)

Fresh beef and veal		
1964	27 lb	12 oz
1974	24 lb	1 oz
1984	20 lb	6 oz
Frozen meat products		
1974	4 lb	6 oz
1984	6 lb	0 oz

Source   National Food Surveys.

The trend is clear, almost exactly what we have lost in fresh meats we have made up in frozen meat products. Frozen burgers alone are worth over £200 million of sales per year to the manufacturers.

The same applies to processed fish products – fish fingers, battered fish, boil-in-the-bag and ready fish meals – compared with fresh, white fish. The trend again is away from fresh fish towards the various forms of frozen processed products (Table 1.2).

Table 1.2
(amount per person per year)

Fresh white fish		
1964	6 lb	12 oz
1974	4 lb	2 oz
1984	3 lb	7 oz
Frozen fish products		
1974	2 lb	3 oz
1984	3 lb	5 oz

Source   National Food Surveys.

Fish fingers alone are worth around £100 million per year to the manufacturers. But – as we shall see later – as the sales of these frozen meat and fish products have been soaring, their quality has not, and their value to our health is being increasingly questioned.

Let us take one further look in the freezer and ask about that favourite treat at pudding time, ice cream. We used to eat most of our ice cream in the street or in a café, and we still eat a lot of it there – over 500 million ice creams each year. But in the last ten years we have more than doubled the amount we eat served at home (Table 1.3).

Table 1.3
(amount per person per year)

Ice cream served at home		
1964	1 lb	12 oz
1974	4 lb	0 oz
1984	9 lb	10 oz

Source   National Food Surveys.

Sales of ice cream are worth over £500 million annually, and the larger ice cream manufacturers spend £5 million on advertising, to get us to buy more.

What else has been happening over the last few decades? Have our main staples of bread and potatoes been affected? Amazingly, despite recent evidence that we are starting to eat more wholemeal bread again after years of decline, the overall consumption of bread has fallen enormously – we now eat only about *half* of what we ate a generation ago. Fresh potatoes, too have seen a similar sharp decline in consumption over the last few decades. And even that old favourite of British breakfasts, porridge oats, has lost two-thirds of its customers since the 1950s (Table 1.4).

Table 1.4
(*amount per person per year*)

Oats and oat products		
1950	4 lb	5 oz
1964	3 lb	2 oz
1974	1 lb	12 oz
1984	1 lb	6 oz

Source   National Food Surveys.

And what has come to replace these staple foods? In the case of porridge oats, the picture is simple: breakfast cereals, which have trebled their consumption as oats have declined (Table 1.5).

Table 1.5
(*amount per person per year*)

Breakfast cereals		
1950	4 lb	9 oz
1964	6 lb	9 oz
1974	9 lb	6 oz
1984	13 lb	7 oz

Source   National Food Surveys.

In the case of potatoes, we now eat more chips, including frozen chips, and crisps than ever before. Frozen chips have rocketed in just ten years, and crisps have increased fivefold in twenty years (Table 1.6).

Table 1.6
(amount per person per year)

	Frozen potato chips	
1974	1 lb	14 oz
1984	6 lb	1 oz
	Crisps and potato snacks	
1964		9 oz
1974	1 lb	13 oz
1984	2 lb	15 oz

Source   National Food Surveys.

Crisps and other 'bag snacks' (i.e. savoury snacks and nuts) have proved very popular. We buy over 5 billion packets each year in Britain. We also buy over 3 billion packets of biscuits!

Most of these figures come from government surveys of what we eat at home. They don't pick up much of the detail on sales of things we eat outside the home, like confectionary and soft drinks. One estimate of what has been happening on the confectionary front is to look at our manufacturing figures (Table 1.7). They aren't exactly accurate as we export some of our sweets and chocolates, and we also import some too – and recently we have imported more chocolate confectionery than we exported, for the first time ever. But total production figures give a fairly clear picture of how our tastes are changing.

Table 1.7
(millions of kilos)

Sweets and confectionery	
1950	401
1964	635
1974	798
1984	802

Source   MAFF/CSO.

A very similar story can be told for soft drinks (Table 1.8). We don't import a great deal of these – most of the 'foreign' names are made under licence in Britain – and we don't export a large amount. The total production figures show a remarkable growth.

Table 1.8
(billions of litres)

	Soft Drinks
1954	1038
1964	2241
1974	3861
1984	5700

Source   MAFF/CSO.

Another clue to our changing diets can be given by the enormous expansion in the use of added ingredients put into processed foods, especially the additives used for making unattractive foods more attractive; the *cosmetic* additives such as the colours, flavours and flavour enhancers. At the beginning of this century about fifty different chemicals were being used in our foods, to preserve the food, to colour it, and to hide the poor quality. Now nearly four thousand different additives are being used in our foods, with nearly a hundred different functions, such as bleaches, solvents, carriers of other additives, foam-reducing agents, emulsifiers, thickeners, sequestrants, antioxidants ... (Don't worry! We explain a bit more about additives later in the book.)

One estimate of how much goes into our food suggests that the figure is around 200 million kilos of additives every year – four kilos for each person in Britain.

Preservatives – which in some foods can stop food poisoning organisms from growing – accounts for just 2 per cent of all these tons of additives. Most additives are there for 'cosmetic' purposes. They are put into food to change the food and make it appear to be something it isn't. They change the texture, feel, taste, flavour or colour so that we are led to believe that it is a food we might like and want. Without the additives we might prefer not to have the food. We might see more than we should, and start demanding something else, something better.

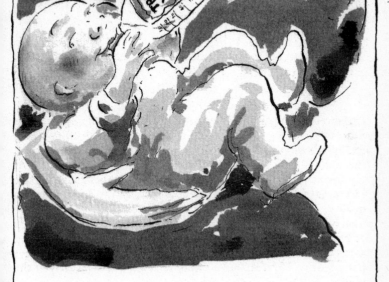

Young Moll has food of mixed repute:
She dines on breast-milk substitute
And every day, on the dot, at six
She shouts and screams to get her fix
Of booze; she causes such a frolic
Her mum will *surely* think it colic,
And with concern give to her daughter
Another slug of pure gripe water.

2 What Are We Being Sold?

So far we have looked at some puzzling, suspicious or alarming things going on in food, which may be worrying if you have to think what on earth to feed your child tonight. Be prepared, because this chapter is quite alarming, too. It takes a closer look at what is going on in the marketing and promotion of children's food, and whether the products really live up to our expectations and our children's needs. *The companies are usually concerned to present themselves in a good light, while in this book we are deliberately taking the opposite view to try to balance things a little.*

But to be quite even handed, we must first of all make a few points:

(a) In being critical of various products we are not trying to single them out as especially bad, but to show that they represent the current trends in practice, and that there may be less bad examples (and maybe some even worse examples).

(b) Very few of the products would do any immediate and specific damage to the average child, and, on the contrary, most of them can provide some very useful nutrients. Our purpose in criticising them is to say: they may be good but they are not as good as they could be. Foods like these can be useful but what we need, and our children deserve, is something better than we are getting. The book is deliberately designed to take a 'critical consumer' approach, always demanding improvements in what is being offered. Any manufacturer with an eye to the future should welcome such criticism as a spur to produce new products to satisfy such demands.

(c) Not everything in this book is negative. Later chapters will look at how we can teach ourselves to be 'critical consumers' by looking carefully at the labels – asking what the words mean and what they might not be saying which they should.

We shall also look at how you can approach nurseries, playgroups and schools with a view to getting changes made for children in groups, and we shall look at how to make a fuss by writing letters and making your views known where it matters – among the senior company staff who are responsible for the products offered in the shops, and among the civil servants and politicians who set the regulations.

But first, we need to take a close and critical look at the sort of products we are being sold today.

THE BABY MARKET

The makers of baby foods have never known such good times. Sales of their products for the tiniest of mouths currently exceed more than £150 million annually.

We are now buying an estimated £60–70 million-worth of baby milk, over £70 million-worth of baby meals in jars and packets, over £14 million-worth of baby drinks and over £10 million-worth of baby rusks every year.

This is a lot of food sales for very tiny appetites. As there are less than 700,000 babies born in Britain in a year, then each one will, on average, have *over £200 spent on buying such tasty delights annually*. Some babies eat much less than this quantity of commercial baby foods – they eat few rusks, don't use formula and rarely get their dinners from jars and packets – which means that many *other* babies are getting a lot more than £200-worth of processed baby-food products into their tiny mouths.

What is happening? What are the reasons for these changes in babies' eating habits and the growing markets for baby milks, drinks and meals.

One reason is *time*. The proportion of women staying at home has halved in the last fifteen years, while the number going out to work (mainly part-time work) has risen by over a million. At the same time, the child-care facilities and support services available have not been growing to meet these needs. The effect can be to reduce the opportunities for a child to have its meals carefully prepared from fresh ingredients. Under pressure, a parent needs food for a baby that is quick to prepare and easy to serve.

A second reason for the growing market in baby food products is a parent's *lack of confidence* and certainty about what is right and healthy for a child, and the subsequent need to rely on the 'authority' of a manufactured product. With all the concerns about healthy diets and the changing advice that experts give about children's needs, anyone having to care for a baby may well feel that they need a qualification in advanced dietetics if they are to cope with it all.

But if they buy a company's 'new, all-natural, vitamin-enriched' brand from a well-known manufacturer then they can assure themselves that they must be doing the right thing. *'It must be all right or it couldn't be sold, could it ...?'* Opening the packet brings instant relief from the anxiety about what is right and wrong for a baby.

One might suspect that it is in the manufacturers' interests to encourage the confusion about what is right and wrong, as they clearly benefit from the resulting anxiety and guilt. Whether or not manufacturers help to feed this anxiety, they certainly make sure they are seen to offer relief. Their labels give long lists of nutrients and have their freedom-from-additives flashed across them (even when the additives are not permitted in the first place). Their promotional literature emphasises their scientific credentials, and shows pictures of marvellously healthy babies in wonderfully wealthy homes, swallowing the product. All this is designed to be, and for many people is, very reassuring.

Which brings us to the third reason for the rising sales in baby foods: the advertising and promotion of these products by the companies concerned. Here are some figures spent by industry on the promotion of baby foods, and for comparison we have shown the figure spent by the government-funded Health Education Council on the promotion of a national healthy eating campaign for people of all ages:

Table 2.1 Corporate promotion

Latest available figures for advertising expenditure on baby foods compared with the Health Education Council's total budget for promoting healthy eating amongst the whole population.

	£
Boots	282,000 (1985)
Cow & Gate	620,000 (1986)
Farley	1,380,000 (1986)
Heinz	760,000 (1986)

Table 2.1 *continued*

Milupa	320,000 (1986)
Robinsons	464,000 (1984)
Wyeth	140,000 (1986)
Other brands	190,000 (1986)
TOTAL	4,156,000
HEC Healthy Eating budget	750,000 (1985)

Sources   Industry data; *British Dental Journal*, 5 July 1986.

BABY'S FIRST TASTE OF COMMERCE

Suppose you worked for a food company and it was your job as a salesman or saleswoman of processed foods to try to get mothers to give up using a common, cheap, easily obtained wholesome food and use your company's special brand of processed food instead. How will you persuade mothers to use it?

Here are some good ideas:

MARKETING METHODS

Method 1   Get it endorsed by important people:

- get leading child experts to say it is OK
- get it approved for use in, say, hospitals or nurseries

Method 2   Give it an image of superiority:

- give some scientific–sounding credentials
- show pictures of affluent people using it
- cast doubts on the older, cheaper, food

Method 3   Give out free samples:

- give out coupons so mothers can collect samples at shops
- best of all, get a professional health worker to give out free samples to each mother.

Method 4   Get advertising literature into authoritative places:

- get it into pharmacies and chemists, rather than grocers
- best is to get it into mother-and-baby clinics
- try and get the health workers to give it to the mothers
- get posters put up in the clinic

Method 5   Appear benevolent:

- give equipment to hospitals
- give free donations of your product to hospitals
- give free gifts to health workers
- sponsor prizes for competitions for beautiful babies
- sponsor awards to health workers who do good works

Method 6   Appear respectable:

- sponsor scientific conferences
- pay some of the costs of health professionals' annual meet-ings, such as a paediatricians' yearly gathering
- have your staff give lectures to health workers at their in-service courses and conferences
- offer counselling services from company advisers

Method 7   Catch them early:

- get your product with its name clearly visible into a mother's hands as soon as it's realistically possible
- get your product into the maternity ward if you can

Method 8   Look responsible:

- agree to restrict 'unethical' promotion practices
- agree on a *Code of Conduct* with your competitors
- agree to set up a committee (on which you sit) to monitor this Code of Conduct

Method 9   Spread it about:

- remember that mothers will be your customers for just a few months, and you would do better spending your promotional budget on winning sympathy from health workers who can speak well of you to thousands of mothers over many years.
- you can be especially friendly to health workers by offering them a few handy little perks, for example:

Diaries	Free conferences
Travel clubs	Free posters
Travel Consultants	Free information packs
Reduced cost flights	Free newsletters and booklets
Magazines to give to mothers	Free samples
Free lunches	Free 'scientific' reports

Sponsored prizes   Pens, note-pads, calendars
Grants for scholarships   Local 'advisers'

And this is exactly what happens. The clearest example is commercial baby milk – infant formula – which the manufacturers want to sell in place of traditional breast-feeding, but the same applies to the commercial weaning food manufacturers. Virtually every one of these practices is actually happening today, with the large baby food and baby milk companies promoting their products just as we have described it, point by point, method by method.

PLEASE NOTE: We are *not* saying that bottle-feeding is *wrong* nor that a woman should feel guilty if she chooses to bottle-feed after hearing the facts and considering her own needs. But we *are* saying that the sort of promotion and marketing practices used by infant formula manufacturers are rarely in the woman's or the child's best interest, and that a mother who ends up bottle-feeding when she didn't intend to should feel angry – angry at the health workers who have failed to support her enough, and angry at the manufacturers who are working so hard to undermine her.

Most mothers, particularly if they have given birth in a British hospital, will be familiar with these bottles (Fig 2.1), or something similar:

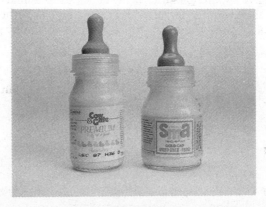

Figure 2.1

They are provided by the manufacturers at cost price, subsidised price or even free to the NHS, and they may be liberally distributed around the maternity wards and the night-time nurseries. The labels state the name of the product in large writing, and carry *none* of the warnings about the hazards of feeding infant formula that is normally required on similar products sold in shops.

Once a baby has been fed on infant formula it may be less hungry when it is next breast-fed. It will want less from the breast. After several occasions of demanding less from the breast, the mother's breast-milk supply will begin to decline. Once the milk starts to decline, the baby will be hungrier at the end of a breast-feed, and the temptation is to give it another bottle.

The downward spiral is easily begun. It is perhaps not surprising that a third of all babies who started off breast-feeding have stopped receiving any breast-milk by the age of one week in Britain. And it is a tragic fact that the longer a mother and baby stay in hospital, where these ready-made commercial bottles are freely available, the more they are likely to give up breast-feeding.

Can we ever replace breast-milk? Companies have been trying to match the composition of breast-milk for years, always hoping to get as 'close to mother's milk' as possible – and actually imply that they are 'closest to mother's milk' in their advertising literature. (They are unlikely ever to match breast-milk, as it will be virtually impossible to match the 'live' immunological elements in breast-milk.) Here is a short history of infant nutrition, in which the baby has often been put in the role of being the scientific guinea pig.

1870s   low-priced condensed milk very popular, but led to increase in scurvy and rickets in infants

1920s   Vitamin A deficiency in infant feeds recognised as cause of xeropthalmia (night blindness)

1928   realisation that copper was essential in infant diets

1950   excess phosphorous in infant feeds was leading to convulsions due to hypocalcaemia

1950   lack of folic acid and Vitamin C in infant feeds was leading to megaloblastic anaemia

1952   data published showing Vitamin A deficiency in infant feeds led to diarrhoea and facial paralysis

1953   molybdenum found to be essential in infant diets

1954   pyridoxine deficiency in infant feeds was leading to fits, cerebral palsy and retardation

1957   data published suggesting excess Vitamin D in infant feeds was leading to hypercalcaemia and kidney damage

1957   selenium found to be essential in infant diets

1958   data published suggesting essential fatty acid deficiency in infant feeds was leading to skin and eye disorders

1959   chromium found to be essential in infant diets

1970   tin found to be essential in infant diets

1971   vanadium found to be essential in infant diets

1972   silicon found to be essential in infant diets

1973   nickel found to be essential in infant diets

1974   National Dried Milk withdrawn due to excess sodium and phosphorus

1976   Vitamin E deficiency in infant feeds may lead to haemolytic anaemia

1977   zinc deficiency in infant feeds suggested as cause of retardation, failure to thrive, and skin disorders

1981   suggestion that hypocalcaemic fits occurred only in young infants fed formula milks

1981   suggestion that hypomagnesaemic fits occurred only in young infants fed formula milks

1981   data published suggesting exess iron in infant feeds may cause bleeding, anaemia and immunological disorders

1982   data published suggesting deficiency of lactobezoars in infant formula causes bowel obstruction

1982   data published suggesting higher rate of necrotising enterocolitis among infants fed on infant formula

1984   neonatal metabolic alkalosis suggested to occur in young infants fed on infant formula

1985   data published showing cases of tetany and hyperparathyroidism in infants fed humanised cow's milk formula

1986   data published suggesting that iron-fortified formula could impair a baby's ability to absorb essential copper

And here is a recent history of specific commercial baby milk products that ran into trouble (partly adapted from Maureen Minchin's book *Breastfeeding Matters*):

1978   *Enfamil with iron* was contaminated with E coli bacteria
1979   *SMA* recalled because improper production has led to gastro-intestinal upsets
1979   *Neo-Mull-Soy* and *Cho-free* found to be deficient in chloride and causing metabolic alkalosis
1980   *Soy-a-lac* and *I-Soy-a-lac* contained excess Vitamin D
1980   *Enfamil with iron* recalled because of curdling and contamination
1981   *Enfamil with iron* recalled because of solvent contamination
1982   Over 2 million cans of *SMA* and *Nursoy* recalled because of Vitamin B6 deficiency
1982   Two cases of contaminated *SMA* concentrate found
1983   *Soy-a-lac* recalled because of unstable Vitamin A
1983   *Naturlac* recalled because deficient in thiamine, copper, and Vitamin B6
1984   *Neo-Ag-U* deficient in calcium, causing tetany
1984   Ready-made *Enfamil* found to be contaminated with E cloacae
1985   Recall of *Kama-Mil* and *Natura-Milk* for various deficiencies, including folates, zinc and Vitamin D
1985   Latex teats used on baby milk bottles suspected of leaking a cancer-causing agent (nitrosamine)
1986   Farley's *Ostermilk* production line closed after forty-one babies suffered salmonella poisoning
1986   Silicon teats used on baby milk bottles and dummies suspected of fragmenting and causing choking – the dummies were withdrawn from sale in the UK.

TRADE TACTICS – BE YOUR OWN JUDGE AND JURY?

Something we cannot show you, because they have produced no public reports or other documents, is the work of the *Code Monitoring Committee*, set up to monitor the Code of Marketing of Breast-Milk Substitutes which the manufacturers wrote in 1983. This code, endorsed by the government, gives the manufacturers a licence to promote their products through the NHS, to give presents to health workers, to advertise to mothers through material given out by health workers, to give free samples to mothers (again through the NHS), and to let sales representatives counsel or visit mothers in hospital wards. All these practices have been condemned by the World Health Organisation.

In 1979, a joint committee of doctors, manufacturers, voluntary agencies, government representatives, officials from UNICEF and the World Health Organisation (WHO) drafted an *International Code of Marketing of Breast-Milk Substitutes* which prohibited all these practices, and at the World Health Assembly in 1981 the UK government, along with 117 other nations, signed a resolution accepting this code. Two years later the UK government allowed the manufacturers to draft a new code without these prohibitions, and it is only this new UK code which is monitored by the Code Monitoring Committee. As if this wasn't weak enough, the Committee:

- does not actively monitor or investigate health service facilities, but depends on receiving complaints;
- is housed in the food manufacturers' (Food and Drink Federation) headquarters;
- has its running costs – the secretary, telephone and other costs – paid for by the food manufacturers' federation;
- in its first three years it has published no report of its work;
- the committee membership includes all four baby milk manufacturers in Britain, and all the other members can only be appointed 'in consultation' with the Food and Drink Federation.

It has been described as a watch-dog with no teeth, that never barks and is fed by the people it is supposed to guard against. One lay member has already resigned over its lack of effectiveness. Yet this committee is supposed to be protecting mothers and babies from undue pressure exerted by manufacturers – just the pressure that the World Health Organisation felt needed to be brought under strict control.

So, should a mother feel guilty if she ends up bottle-feeding when she intended to breast-feed? Of course not. But angry? *Yes!*

TRADE TACTICS – A LITTLE FRIGHTENER

Once upon a time, breast-feeding was a matter of putting a baby to a breast. Sometimes a little help and encouragement was needed, sometimes a hand from someone more experienced was useful, at least to get started.

Then various companies, including those already making bottles for formula feeding, hit on a bright idea. Why not make the whole thing so complicated and terrifying that no mother in her right mind would try it, or if she did it would cost her dearly. How would a company set about this task? Here are the tips:

- start by reminding women how often there may be problems;
- suggest that continuing to breast-feed sometimes needs 'determination' and 'perseverance';
- show pictures of women breast-feeding – but make these quite unattractive, e.g. with the woman stripped to the waist or even totally naked;
- give a few details of how a baby is totally dependent on the one person – unless the mother expresses milk or uses formula;
- do not imply that breast-milk can be expressed by hand, but indicate the machinery you could (and should) use;
- expressing milk should not look easy – give detailed instructions on how to sterilise the pumps and use the milk;
- make the breast pumps look ugly, and make them look complicated high-tech machines, and make them expensive.

Here are some examples from the literature (Fig. 2.2) produced by the companies who are aiming at the 'breast-feeder' market:

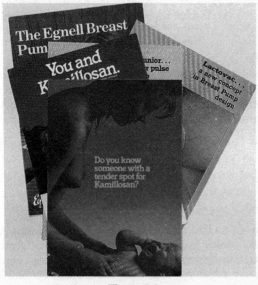

Figure 2.2

BABY DRINKS

By about 4–6 months most babies will be starting to try 'solid' foods. Although there are no biological reasons for cutting back on breast-milk as the main drink, even after a year, there are often practical reasons why a baby will be offered other drinks instead. In principle, water is all that is actually needed if the baby is still getting breast-milk or formula, and is starting to eat a variety of foods.

Water may be all a child actually needs, but food companies wouldn't make much money offering you bottles of plain water. They need us to think that water 'may not be enough' and we should buy products which are 'enriched' in some way.

Dietitians usually suggest weaning on to cow's milk after the baby has passed the six-month point, or else continuing on breast-milk or formula milk. Only if the baby is refusing to eat a varied range of foods would there be any need to find ways of providing additional nutrition through the drinks. But if cow's milk is to be used there are a few drawbacks that are sometimes raised, and manufacturers have not been slow to offer alternatives:

- for a small number of children, cow's milk is not tolerated well, and can induce allergies such as asthma and eczema;
- cow's milk has less Vitamin C than breast-milk or infant formula;
- cow's milk – especially full-cream milk – is higher in saturated fats and lower in polyunsaturated fats than breast-milk or formula milk, with possible consequences for the child's health in the long term;
- cow's milk is not a good source of iron.

As a result of these drawbacks with cow's milk we can now find on the shelves of the chemists and supermarkets a range of apparent solutions, none of which is particularly cheap.

Goat's milk and soya milk

Goat's milk is offered as an alternative to cow's milk, on the basis that it has different characteristics and so may be better tolerated. What little hard evidence there is suggests that goat's milk offers no substantial advantages to cow's milk-intolerant children, but some parents may find it useful. Remember that it costs more, it is even richer in saturated fats than cow's milk and has low levels of vital folic acid. Otherwise it is similar to cow's milk. Check that it has been pasteurised as there have been instances of goat's milk not being pasteurised before use. A young child could get a serious dose of food poisoning or other infectious disease from such non-pasteurised milk.

Soya milk comes in two forms – as a simple milk *drink* made from soya beans, and as a carefully made up *formula* using soya milk as the base instead of cow's milk. This second product is designed as a substitute for bottle-feeding children in their first few months, rather than as a drink in later months. It's composition is designed to be equivalent to that of the other formula milks, and the main difference from most families' viewpoint will be the extra cost. A month's supply of soya-formula milk costs around £18–£30 compared with £15–£20 for a month's supply of regular formula milk, and the obviously lower costs of breast-milk.

At least two manufacturers currently market soya-based formula feeds. These forms of infant formula are the preferred variety for vegans and others who want their children to eat no animal products but are not breast-feeding. Yet one manufacturer, Wyeth, actually puts animal fat (beef fat or lard) into the soya formula, making it quite unacceptable for these families.

Soya milk drinks, on the other hand, should not be used to replace formula milks or breast-milks, but are offered as a substitute for cow's milk for an older baby or anyone else. If someone is genuinely cow's milk intolerant, or if you object to using cow's milk for some reason, then there may be some point in trying a product like this provided you don't mind paying. It costs around 35p–40p per pint, compared with regular milk at 27p or less per pint.

For a child who is getting a variety of foods, with care taken to ensure that the nutritional benefits of milk are made available in other forms, then neither cow's milk nor soya milk need be used.

Follow-ups

To cater for the anxiety that the saturated fats in cow's milk might create in a worried child-carer, one manufacturer has marketed a *follow-up milk drink* designed to be used after a baby has reached its sixth month. Despite its presentation in packs similar to the infant formula packs, it is *not* a substitute for breast-milk or formula. Initially, the manufacturers were trying to persuade mothers to start using their product for babies of four months, but the DHSS – after some angry letters from health workers – asked the manufacturers to change their 'suitable from four months' claim to 'not suitable before six months'.

The product is sold mainly on its lower concentration of saturated fats compared with cow's milk. Although this may be the case, it still does not conform with the requirements of a World Health Organisation expert committee, who stated that any milk for babies should have various essential polyunsaturated fatty acids present to match those that can be found in breast-milk and which are considered essential in the optimum development of nerve and brain cells, veins and arteries. One professor of nutrition has examined the nutrients used in the follow-on milk and said that the balance of fats and other nutrients were suitable for mammals that needed to put on a lot of weight in a short time. The follow-up milk product was, he said, suitable for feeding to a young rhinoceros.

TRADE TACTICS – TELLING SOME PORKY PIES

The company making this product has claimed in correspondence with the London Food Commission that it has the support of experts in various eminent organisations. It claimed its product was

> based on recommendations for 'follow on' formula milks put out by the WHO, EEC, and European Society for Gastroenterology and Nutrition. All of these recommended the use of follow on formulas from 4–6 months onwards.
>
> Letter to *LFC*, 13.6.1986

So we wrote to these organisations and asked if they did indeed endorse the use of follow-on milks for young children, either before or after 6 months of age.

It turns out that the last of the three organisations, known as ESPGAN and reputed to have close links with food companies, recommended 'the replacement of the starting formula by a *less expensive* follow-up formula' from the age of 4–6 months (our italics).

The EEC includes follow-up milks in their proposed legislation on infant formula, but these proposals do not endorse the use of follow-up milk so much as *restrict* its promotion and marketing. And the WHO (World Health Organisation) had, at their thirty-ninth World Health Assembly just a month before the company wrote their letter to the London Food Commission, published a statement about feeding young children. It included the following declaration:

> The practice being introduced in some countries of providing infants with specially formulated milks (so-called 'follow-up' milks) is not necessary.
>
> Item 21, WHA 30.28 (16.5.86)

Some health workers have been very critical of the company producing this follow-on milk drink, particularly as it can appear to replace the use of a formula milk. The very phrase 'follow-up' milk might be taken to imply that it is something a baby should transfer onto after a few months on an infant formula, as a full replacement for that formula. The manufacturers themselves promote it as 'the next step'. But it is *not* adequate nutrition on its own. As it usually costs more than regular formula, and more than regular cow's milk – and is more hazardous to prepare than cow's milk – there seems little justification for its use.

The latest DHSS recommendations on infant nutrition advise using breast-milk or infant formula up to the age of one year, after which cow's milk is suitable. If cow's milk is being used between 6 months and a year, then, according to the DHSS, follow-up milks have one advantage: they offer 'a more reliable source of Vitamin D and iron'. But as no one should expect milk to be the main source of iron in a child's diet, and as Vitamin D is available in other foods, in the vitamin drops supplied at low cost from baby clinics, and can be made by the body when exposed to sunshine, there may seem little to gain from replacing doorstep milk with this sort of commercial follow-up milk drink.

Vitamin C at all costs?

One anxiety which a parent may have is whether their baby is getting enough Vitamin C. Welfare orange juice used to be sold at baby clinics as a means of ensuring that no baby was short of Vitamin C in their diet, and nowadays the same approach is taken by offering the low-cost vitamin drops that are recommended by health visitors and available from baby clinics.

A good diet can provide all the Vitamin C needed, and along with the vitamin drops there should be no reason for a child to go short of sufficient Vitamin C for their daily needs. Yet manufacturers fall over themselves to offer Vitamin C enriched drinks as if they were essential.

Cow's milk is not a rich source of Vitamin C and should not be relied on as the main source in an older baby's diet. For a 1-year-old, a pint of fresh cow's milk can provide a third of the recommended Vitamin C for the day. If the child is also eating some fresh fruit and vegetables, including potatoes, then they are unlikely to suffer scurvy, the main symptom of Vitamin C deficiency.

We do not know whether manufacturing Vitamin C synthetically and putting it into sweet drinks for a baby to suck on is going to do as much good as offering Vitamin C in its original form – in the fruit, vegetables and milk which can provide it. Producing sweet, fruit-flavoured water, with added Vitamin C synthesised in laboratories, can be questioned as to its value to a child. There is little doubt as to its value to the manufacturers, who have realised that Vitamin C acts as a preservative and antioxodant, keeping the product from deteriorating over long periods and stopping the colour from fading – while at the same time they can suggest to us they have done our children a nutritional favour.

Some bad publicity on the Esther Ranzen TV show exposed the potential danger of giving sweet syrupy so-called 'health' drinks in bottle-feeders. The syrup was accused of giving children a sweet tooth, and also giving them many rotten ones. The publicity fell mostly on the rose-hip syrups and the blackcurrant syrups, both cases where the purchaser was being sold Vitamin C as the reason for buying the product, and getting an enormous load of sugar thrown in besides.

So what are we offered now? Drinks with no sugar? Don't you believe it! Every one of the drinks listed below is sweet-tasting. Everyone can, potentially, encourage tooth decay.

And every one can replace a portion of the child's needs for nutrient-rich calories.

The University of Leeds Dental Health Department have reported recently that the numbers of children referred to their clinic with 'rampant dental caries of the primary incisors and molars' (which is typical of 'nursing bottle caries') did not seem to be falling. In a recent letter to the medical journal, *The Lancet*, the University said they felt it was important to examine the products now being sold to mothers who are trying to reduce the risk of tooth decay.

When the researchers analysed some examples (Table 2.2) they found that every one that they looked at had sugars in one form or another. Even if it was not in the form of sucrose it could, they said, 'Demineralise tooth enamel just as much as sucrose-based drinks'.

Table 2.2
Weaning onto soft drinks

Drink	Teaspoons of sugar*
Robinson's apple/cherry	4.1
Robinson's apple/plum/orange	4.1
Cow & Gate pear/peach	3.9
Cow & Gate apple/blackcurrant	3.5
Robinson's apple/orange	3.3
Delrosa apple/cherry	2.4
Delrosa apple/blackcurrant	2.4
Delrosa apple/orange	2.3
Cow & Gate summer fruits	2.2
Beecham's Baby Ribena orange	2.0
Beecham's Baby Ribena	1.9
Robinson's apple/blackcurrant	1.5

* the teaspoon equivalent of sucrose.
Source Curzon *et al.*, *The Lancet*, 5.3.88.

From the teeth's point of view, the actual quantity of sugars is less important than the fact that they are there at all. Most of the sugar will be swallowed, and it is principally the time that the sugar is in contact with the teeth, all by itself, that matters most. Feeding bottles are one of the slowest, and so most prolonged, ways of drinking these products, and a feeding cup would be better. The university dentists recommended that if these drinks were to be used then they should only be provided at meal times, and that drinks between meals should be milk (without sugar added) or water. Fruit juice is not usually recommended by dentists, as the acid in the juice can act with the natural sugars present to attack the teeth, even if the juice is diluted.

The suggestions that the syrup-based baby drinks can be tooth-damaging, and that because of the sugar they should be best served during meals, are rarely made on the packets, and never in big print. Quite the opposite. Here are some of the labels (Fig. 2.3) put on just the products that were analysed by the University of Leeds:

LOW IN ACIDITY

NO ADDED SUGAR

NO PRESERVATIVES

NO ARTIFICIAL COLOURS

NO ARTIFICIAL FLAVOURS

NO ARTIFICIAL SWEETENERS

NO ADDED SUGAR

NO ARTIFICIAL SWEETENER

NO ARTIFICIAL FLAVOURING

NO ARTIFICIAL COLOURING

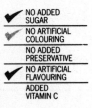

NO ADDED SUGAR

NO ARTIFICIAL COLOURING

NO ADDED PRESERVATIVE

NO ARTIFICIAL FLAVOURING

ADDED VITAMIN C

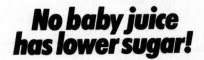

No baby juice has lower sugar!

Figure 2.3

Colicky baby? – turn to the booze

Some babies, especially during the first three months, seem prone to develop colic – typically crying and not settling easily and appearing to be in pain. There is some evidence linking colic to cow's milk – either in the baby's bottle-feed or, if the baby breast-feeds, in the mother's diet.

The harassed parents of a colicky child will do anything if they think it might cure the child's problem, and give both the child and the parent a peaceful break. Manufacturers have not missed this opportunity (Fig. 2.4).

The safe, gentle way of relieving baby's wind, quickly eases hiccups and minor tummy upsets. Woodward's Gripe Water has been famous for over 100 years as a safe and gentle method of relieving wind pains and minor tummy upsets in babies and young children, particularly at the difficult period when they are cutting teeth.

Gripe Mixture

Nurse Harvey's after a feed soothes away wind, tummy pain and colic. It is a great comfort during teething. Baby sleeps soundly at night and you get the rest you need to restore your energy.

Soothing, settling, gentle

Its balanced formula and gentle action make Dinneford's ideal for bringing up painful wind and settling tummy upsets so that both baby and mother may enjoy essential rest and sleep. The Mixture also effectively relieves colic pains, checks hiccups and eases difficult motions. It will,

Figure 2.4

One 'traditional' remedy is Gripe Water. Whether it has an effect on the colic or not is a matter of some dispute. Manufacturers say that it can be effective in relieving colic, settling a stomach and easing wind – but many health workers are dubious of these claims. What is certain is that it can have an effect on the symptoms of pain through a very simple mechanism: namely, getting the baby tanked up on alcohol. Just look at the ingredients in Table 2.3:

Table 2.3 A drop of the hard stuff?

Dinneford's Gripe Mixture:	
Magnesium carbonate	2%
Citric acid	4%
Sodium bicarbonate	2%
Sugar	25%
Alcohol	5%
Woodward's Gripe Water:	
Dill water	4%
Sodium bicarbonate	1%
Ginger tincture	1%
Syrup	15%
Alcohol	5%
Nurse Harvey's Gripe Mixture:	
Dill and caraway oils	0.1%
Sodium bicarbonate	1%
Syrup	20%
Ginger tincture	5%

(And in case you are thinking that Nurse Harvey uses no alcohol, remember that ginger tincture is 150° proof spirit.)
Source   Packet labels.

There is pure alcohol, up to 5 per cent pure alcohol, in these mixtures. The strength is higher than many commercial lagers and beers, and the recommended dose for a baby of 2 months (10ml) can be, weight for weight, equal to an adult drinking half of a measure of gin. According to the manufacturers, this sort of dose can be given up to eight times in a day. For a small body that has never experienced an alcoholic drink the result could be quite stupefying.

Gripe waters are also rich in syrup, which along with the alcohol provides calories with virtually no useful nutrients. The daily amounts suggested for a baby of 2 months could give the baby as much as 80 calories, or 6–7 per cent of its daily need, while giving none of the normal nutrients a growing body requires.

Herbal teas – or market tease?

Based on the unproven suggestion that fennel, a relative of cow-parsley and hog-weed, may settle a baby's upset stomach, and making reference to the herbal teas used in Asia, one baby food company has started promoting a fennel drink which is largely sweetened water. A commercial drink like this is not a traditional herbal tea. It has been promoted with free sachets in the Bounty Bags and Treasure Trove gift packs handed out by health workers in the maternity wards and baby clinics, and on the counters of chemists' shops.

The amount of actual fennel in these drinks is minute – less than 5 per cent in the sachet – and there is no certainty that the active ingredient (if there is one) is still in the fennel after it has been through the various processes to end up in the sachets.

What is in the sachet? The answer is well over 90 per cent by weight dextrose, a type of sugar. Made up as instructed, the drink is nearly as sweet as Cola. Plain sugar costs around 50p per kilo, but this form of dextrose works out around £4–5 for the weight of a one-kilo bag.

The drink is sold as suitable for babies 'from around weaning age'. Many health professionals are appalled at its promotion as a suitable drink for such young children. The company urges parents not to use the drink to replace a baby's regular breast- or bottle-feed, and yet the empty calories provided in this drink inevitably replace calories from other, more nutritious sources. Soft drinks instead of nutrition?

Dentists have become alarmed at the potential damage that starting a child on soft drinks can do to the newly developing teeth. A company manufacturing the sweetened 'tea' drink were sued in West Germany by a mother who claimed that her child's teeth were damaged by the use of this product. The company – presumably fearing the bad publicity that a public trial might bring – offered to settle out of court, for a figure understood to be around DM40,000 (about £12,000).

Understandably, rather than face a court hearing and further legal wrangling, the mother agreed to drop the case. If the company had been found in court to be liable for damaging the child's teeth then this would have been the first such case of its kind in Europe, and a strong precedent for consumer action against these sorts of products.

A final word on milk for infants

Once the only cow's milk available came direct from the cow. It was boiled before serving to babies. Now there are over a dozen different sorts of milk available in the grocers, with little indication of which might be most suitable for young children.

This is what we found in a grocery:

Regular full-cream (silver top)
Homogenised full-cream (red top)
Semi-skimmed
Skimmed
Channel island (gold top)
Calcium-enriched (Shape, Calcia)
Banana flavour
Chocolate flavour
Strawberry flavour
Sterilised milk
UHT full-cream
UHT semi-skimmed
UHT skimmed
Soya milk
Powdered milk
Powdered skimmed milk
Coffee whitener (milk substitute)

Only the full-cream milks are currently recommended by the DHSS for young children aged 6 months to 2 years, with semi-skimmed milk an alternative for children over 2 years. There is nothing on any of these milk products to indicate their suitability or non-suitability for young children.

Now, in addition to the long list, we have the new development in the dairy industry of milk produced from cows which have been injected with BST (Bovine Somatotropin). There is some evidence emerging on the effects this might have on the milk itself, and there is plenty of evidence of what effect it can have on the welfare of the cow that produces it.

For the milk, some reports have shown that the levels of fat are increased in the milk from cows injected with BST, by as much as 27 per cent. As milk fat (butterfat) is high in saturated fatty acids, and low in polyunsaturates, this is not a very desirable feature. It is not a health bonus for most young children. But BST milk is not separately labelled. It is being mixed in with the rest of the milk supply, so we have no choice – we will get it whether we want to or not.

For the cows, the advent of BST has meant they are being stimulated by this extra hormone to pump out milk at a rate 10 to 20 per cent above their usual levels. The cows 'burn out' and their milk-producing life is shortened.

We do not *need* BST-produced milk. Whether it will have an impact on our children's health we simply do not know. Only future generations will judge.

FIRST SOLID FOODS

For a child's first experience of solid foods we have for many years been advised by health educators and other professionals to hunt around the shelves full of weaning foods and find that rare commodity *baby rice*. In among the many other competing products, including such tempting ones as 'baby rice pudding', 'baby rice with vegetables, etc.' we may chance to find the real thing. Baby rice is in fact ordinary ground rice, or possibly a finely flaked rice, which may be precooked for instant reconstitution. Only one baby food company seems to sell such a product in its simple form (Milupa). Two other products which promote themselves as a baby's first food are Farley's Farex Rice Based Cereal – with rice, corn, soya and various added vitamins, etc., and Robinson's Baby Rice – which includes various added minerals and vitamins and a sweet flavouring, malt extract.

But the first thing you might notice about baby rice is the price (Table 2.4). It comes in fancy boxes, so you may not immediately realise what it costs per pound weight. In fact, it can set you back anything from £1.40p to £2.50 per lb which does not compare well with the basic ingredient – rice – that can be bought for less than £0.30p per lb in most supermarkets.

Table 2.4 The price of 'rice'

	cost per lb
Milupa pre-cooked rice flakes	1.43p
Robinson's Baby Rice	2.40p
Farley's Farex, rice based cereal	1.74p
Supermarket own label ground rice	30p
Supermarket own label rice flakes	56p
Supermarket own label white rice	28p

Source LFC.

Adding in the vitamins would make sense if the baby is getting few vitamins elsewhere. But if the baby is getting breast-milk, or infant formula, it is unlikely to be going short. And if it is taking its recommended vitamin drops from the baby clinic then that should be more than enough. It won't need the extra. They will mostly go in one end and out the other. The babies who might be going short of vitamins are those needing special diets or those in families where poverty or other factors have led to a poor diet for the baby, which includes insufficient breast-milk or formula milk. In such situations the expensive, fortified baby rice products are not easily afforded and may not be bought.

The main advantage of using rice for young babies is that, unlike wheat, it has no *gluten*, a protein which can cause intolerance reactions in some babies if fed before the age of around 6 months. Dietitians nowadays are suggesting alternatives to cereal foods as the first solids for weaning: puréed potato or puréed dahl, and puréed fruit and vegetables (though these have less calories in each spoonful). All of these are gluten-free and can be used as well as rice.

WEANING BABIES – OR MUMS?

Getting a child's dinner from a packet seems to have become commonplace in many British kitchens, and even for a baby's first taste of solid foot it seems to be increasingly the case that we rely on something instant, rather than mashing the food we ourselves might be eating. In some cultures – perhaps not often found in Britain – it is standard routine to give the baby food from the mother's (or grandmother's) own mouth. It is ready to eat and at just the right temperature!

Feeding a baby from the mother's mouth, or at least her plate, would hardly bring in the billions for the multinationals. They need to convince us that they have better things to offer – in any variety you want.

And convince us they have. When 5,000 mothers of recently weaned babies were asked what foods they had offered their baby the previous day, only 35 per cent said that they had offered something that they had made themselves, while an incredible 82 per cent had offered commercial baby foods.

Dry or wet, in packets or jars, we have never been presented with such a wide variety of possible choices when it comes to giving our babies their dinners. And now we are seeing further 'product diversification' into the realm of non-dinner baby meals: baby breakfasts, baby teas and suppers, to say nothing of the sweet snacks (e.g. rusks) and soft drinks (syrups, juices and herbal drinks) we look at elsewhere.

The shelves of the shops are having to expand to make way for all these products. A whole new range was introduced recently, made by Bebelac in Greece and set up to compete with the market leaders in dry, instant baby meals, Milupa, Robinsons and Boots. Familia is also attacking this market, offering the wholesome Swiss image, and Farley's are trying out a line of packet meals aimed at breakfast-time.

Sales of ready-to-eat jars and tins of baby foods are dominated by the two multinational companies, Cow & Gate and Heinz. Retailer shops' own-label products are also available – Boots, for example, takes a significant slice of the total market.

The range of products for tempting babies – or is it parents? – is large and expanding. Even a small supermarket will offer up to thirty or more varieties of jars and packets. Milupa and Robinsons both list over thirty different baby food meals, and Heinz lists over seventy.

To compete, these products have to offer the harassed shopper some attractive features. Whoever feeds the child must know that the child will want to eat the stuff, that there will be no bad reactions, and that the food will be of some value nutritionally. Knowing that parents have become increasingly concerned about the quality of foods offered by the food industry in this country, baby food manufacturers have jumped at the chance to claim the superiority of their products – their nutritional benefits, their purity, their freedom from additives and so forth.

If manufacturers claim something for their products which is actually untrue then they are breaking the law. In this book we are not in a position to say that any claims made by manufacturers are actually untrue. We have not chemically analysed the products they sell to see whether their claims about additives, say, are honest, or whether the nutritional quality is exactly what they say it is.

TRADE TACTICS – ACCENTUATE THE POSITIVE

For the most part we accept that manufacturers do not intentionally deceive us, the consumers. But we do come across examples of promotional material which border on the misleading. The truth might be told – but not all of it. Claims might be made – but they are left open to interpretation. An absolute statement may be made – but it means little on its own and needs to be put on a usable scale. These are the ways of promoting products and the stuff of commercial business, but their value to consumers can be little or nothing, and occasionally worse than nothing. They appear to be informative when in fact they leave us little the wiser.

In Chapter 3 of this book we will look in more detail at the claims on the labels and what sometimes lies behind them. For the moment, here are some examples of the sorts of 'flash-bands' which feature on many of the products, supposedly giving us useful nutritional information:

Tactic 1   'No added sugar'
Watch out: this could mean other sorts of sweetening are being used, such as concentrated fruit juice or sugar by another name such as glucose, dextrose or maltose. Or else it might be a savoury dish where one would not expect sugar anyway.

Tactic 2   'Low sugar'
Watch out: what they call low can still mean very high, as we find in the case of teething rusks. Remember that *low sugar* means there *is* sugar there, so you might want to avoid it.

Tactic 3   'No artificial sweeteners'
Watch out: artificial sweeteners are banned from baby foods by law. The company is saying it is obeying the law. They are also distracting you from asking whether sugar or some other permitted sweetener has been added – which it usually has.

Tactic 4   'No added colours'
Watch out: added colours are being banned from baby foods by law (apart from three colours which are also vitamins). Again the company is only saying that it is obeying the law.

Tactic 5   'No flavour enhancer'
Watch out: flavour enhancers are banned from baby foods by law. This includes monosodium glutamate. But there are other chemicals which are not listed by the government as 'flavour enhancers'

that can have the same effect of boosting the flavour. Hydrolysed vegetable protein is one that is commonly found in baby foods. It gives a meaty, savoury taste to bland foods – but it is not technically a flavour enhancer.

Tactic 6 'No preservatives'
Watch out: there may be preserving agents present which are not listed by the government as 'preservatives'. Concentrated sugar acts as a preservative, so does Vitamin C, and vinegar, and salt. Or the food may be vacuum wrapped or packed in an inert gas. All this means is that, although you may not be getting a listed preservative, you may well be getting food that is not fresh but has been preserved by other means.

Tactic 7 'Only natural ingredients'
Watch out: the sorts of chemicals being called natural include ones from plants and animals that we would not expect in our diet. They have not all been tested as much as the old-fashioned artificial colours. The word 'natural' can mean chemicals derived from insects, crab shells, bird feathers, seaweed, cotton and wood. And manufacturers can also use chemicals synthesised in laboratories which are *similar* to ones found in nature, and call these 'natural' or 'nature-identical', too.

FOR MORE INFORMATION ON HOW TO READ LABELS, SEE CHAPTER 4.

SMALL DINNERS – BIG DEALS

There are currently two ways in which we can buy an 'instant' meal for our baby from the shop shelves – either as a just-add-water-or-milk dry powder in a packet, or as an open-and-serve, ready-to-eat blended wet food in a jar or tin.

A lightweight packet offering an instant multivitamin dinner for one may be just what every harassed mum-on-the-move needs. Millions of these packs are sold every week. The market is dominated by Robinsons and Milupa, with inroads being made by Farleys, Boots, Bebelac and Familia (Fig. 2.5). Apart from Familia's highly sugared but unfortified muesli, the companies all rely on a similar sort of recipe: take some dried, powdered food, add starches and/or sugars, and garnish with a liberal sprinkling of powdered vitamins and minerals. Nutritionist Caroline Walker described these sorts of baby foods on the BBC Food Programme as 'cardboard with vitamin pills'.

Vitamin A	450 µg
Thiamin	0.5 mg
Riboflavin	0.6 mg
Niacin	7 mg
Vitamin B6	0.9 mg
Folic Acid	100 µg
Vitamin B12	2µg
Vitamin C	60 mg
Vitamin D	10 µg
Calcium	600 mg
Iron	7 mg
Zinc	4mg

INGREDIENTS:

Rice Flour 68% Maize Flour, Soya Flour, Calcium Carbonate, Yeast, Vitamin C, Niacin, Iron, Vitamins A, Thiamin (B$_1$), Riboflavin (B$_2$) and D.

INGREDIENTS

Carrots, Tomatoes, rice flour, Soya flour, Cauliflower, Maltodextrin, Onions, Peas, Minerals (Dicalcium phosphate, Calcium carbonate, Reduced iron). Hydrolysed vegetable protein, Vitamins (Vitamin C, Niacin, Pantothenic acid, Vitamin A, Riboflavin (Vitamin B2), Thiamin (Vitamin B1), Vitamin B6, Folic acid, Biotin, Vitamin D, Vitamin B12).

Ingredients

Whole oat flour, dried skimmed milk with vegetable fat, sugar, maltodextrin, dried full cream milk, glucose, vitamin concentrate containing vitamins C, E, Ca-D-pantothenate, nicotinamide, vitamins A, B$_2$, B$_1$, B$_6$, folic acid, biotin, vitamins D$_3$ and B$_{12}$), vanilla, calcium carbonate, cinnamon, ferric saccharate.

Figure 2.5

For these sorts of foods, the processes involved in cooking the raw ingredients, dehydrating them and grinding them into a fine powder can destroy many of the vitamins that may have been present. This reduction in nutritional quality is made worse by adding substantial amounts of starches and sugars, creating a 'dinner' with plenty of calories but few nutrients.

The mineral and vitamin list might well look rather poor after all this, and compared with fresh home-cooked food (and even compared with the ready-to-eat tins and jars of weaning food) the companies making these packet dinners would be accused of encouraging poor diets and encouraging malnourishment. So into the mix go handfuls of health-promoting nutrients, most of them straight from chemical laboratories. What we end up with is an instant food, bulked out with starches and sugars, and pepped up with a seemingly impressive list of fortifying biochemicals.

The starches and sugars are added for several reasons. For a start, the starch helps pick up the added water or milk, turning the powder into a 'mash' which the baby can eat. The starch swells and softens and holds all the ingredients in a paste for easy spooning and easy chewing.

Babies do not need their own special instant foods. Mashing up what *you* are eating may be all that the baby would need. But if you do want to prepare something instant, without paying quite so much money, then here is a tip. When the baby has passed 6 months and is happily eating bread and other gluten-containing products, then you can forget the baby cereals and use other semi-instant cereals. The main ones, like Ready Brek and the supermarket's own-label loo-kalikes, are usually low in added sugars, free of added highly refined starches and free of added salt. They have a similar sprinkling of vitamins, but cost a whole lot less (Table 2.5).

Table 2.5 Costs of instant meals

Brands		Typical cost per 100g (up to 10 small servings)
Milupa dinners		66p
Robinsons		95p
Familia		41p
Farley (Farex)		40p
Farley (Breakfast Timers)	50p	
Bebelac (Biski crem)	45p	
Boots		85p
Ready Brek		17p
Own-label instant cereal	15p	

Source LFC.

(*Note*: do check the packet first – for example, Ready Brek Country Style *has* got added sugar though regular Ready Brek has not.)

The starches serve another purpose: they can help the manufacturer distribute the product into the packs. The dextrins and maltodextrins are fine powder which flow well, and so are useful to the manufacturer to 'improve the smooth consistency' of their product – i.e. stop the stuff sticking, caking and forming lumps.

Lastly, these ingredients – the starches and sugars – are cheap and help to make up the bulk and weight of the product. With a final price of these baby dinners in the region of £3–4 per pound, and the costs to the manufacturers of an extra vitamin pill in each packet, these sorts of products appear to be highly profitable lines for the companies concerned.

Besides the questionable quality – with the added starches and sugars – and besides the fancy prices, there are some remaining questions about the added vitamins and minerals. Should we pay much attention to them? Do they make everything all right again by providing a complete nutritional substitute for freshly cooked food? Or do they raise any potential problems for a baby?

First, how complete are they? The manufacturers would not dare to claim that their product was really a complete food (only infant formula attempts to compete with breast-milk by trying to satisfy all of a baby's needs, and then only for the first 4–6 months). But these commercial products do give an *impression* that they *might* be complete with various phrases on the packets (Fig. 2.6):

BOOTS BABY FOODS have been specially formulated using pure, wholesome ingredients to provide a nutritious balanced diet for your baby.

- Prepared for babies' taste buds.
- Allows a nutritionally balanced diet.
- Gives satisfying, wholesome nourishment.

Milupa infant food provides balanced, natural nourishment for babies starting on solids and for growing children at any meal time. Introduce

Farex by Farley's is the ideal and natural way to introduce solid foods to your baby. It provides energy and essential nutrients – protein, vitamins and minerals – to help ensur that your baby receives a well-balanced diet.

Figure 2.6

The trouble is, that we do not actually know what complete nutrition is. If you looked at a dictionary at the end of the last century you would not have found the word 'vitamins' at all – the phrase was coined from the words 'vital amines' in 1912. Even by the 1930s you would probably have found only six or so vitamins listed. And as we saw in the section looking at the history of creating infant formula, various essential trace elements and other nutrients were not fully identified till the 1950s and 1960s, and compounds such as polyunsaturated fatty acids are still subject to some debate today.

What supplements are needed? Until the last two decades very few foods could be found with mineral and vitamin fortification. White flour was one, which was fortified during the Second World War and the practice has continued ever since. During the decades that followed babies were not given extracted supplements so much as food products which were rich sources of nutrients – such as orange juice and milk powder. Only in the 1960s were these withdrawn and the baby clinics instructed to offer commercial infant formula and vitamin drops instead. The manufacturers of dried weaning foods picked up the idea of fortification, and by the early 1980s were making a feature of their fortifying lists on the sides of their packs.

But how do these compare with the vitamin supplements you can buy for children in chemists and health food shops? Here are some comparisons (Table 2.6): the first list is that shown on the side of a pack of fortified weaning food, the second list is that given for a brand of children's multivitamin and mineral supplements, and the third list is the ingredients of a home-made purée of plain potato and egg yolk.

The question is, if the processed weaning foods do *not* give complete nutrition, then what is missing? And would the companies like to make it clear where we should get the missing ingredients from? Is the answer 'ordinary food'?

Satisfying a baby's appetite with a processed instant dinner gives it some but not all its nutrients needs, but could lead to it not getting the rest of what it requires. That's the trouble with what nutritionist Caroline Walker has called 'cardboard and vitamin pills'!

Table 2.6   Food or supplements?

Nutrient list from the fortified packs compared with vitamin pills and with a plain home-made dish.

Fortified weaning food	Children's multivitamins	Sieved potato with some egg yolk
Fat	Safflower oil	Fats, including
Protein	and fatty acids	essential linoleic acid
Carbohydrate	Bioflavonoids	linolenic acid
Vitamin A	Vitamin A	arachidonic acid
Vitamin B1	Vitamin B1	Protein, including
Vitamin B2	Vitamin B2	essential isoleucine
Niacin	Niacin	leucine
Vitamin B6	Vitamin B6	lysine
Vitamin B12	Vitamin B12	methionine
Folic acid	Folic acid	cystine
Pantothenic acid	Pantothenic acid	phenylalanine
Biotin	Biotin	tyrosine
Vitamin C	Choline Bitartrate	threonine
Vitamin D	Inositol	tryptophan
Calcium	P-Aminobenzoic acid	valine
Phosphorus	Vitamin C	histidine
Iron	Vitamin E	Vitamin A
	Vitamin D	Vitamin B1
	Vitamin K	Vitamin B2
	Calcium	Niacin
	Magnesium	Vitamin B6
	Chromium	Vitamin B12
	Iron	Folic acid
	Manganese	Pantothenic acid
	Molybdenum	Biotin
	Iodine	Vitamin C
	Copper	Calcium
	Zinc	Magnesium
		Phosphorus
		Iron
		Copper
		Zinc
		Selenium

Sources   Product labels; McCane and Widdowson, *The Composition of Foods*, HMSO, 1985.

The box indicates the sort of added fortification that the processed weaning food-makers put in their packs. We are not able to say what other nutrients may be present, even in tiny, trace amounts, so we simply do not know whether the food is adequate on its own. If it is *not* adequate then there is a danger of entirely satisfying a baby's appetite without satisfying its needs for nutrients.

There is another possibility too. The baby could be getting more than it needs of some nutrients. By feeding a baby with fortified foods, ultra-rich in some nutrients, as well as continuing with, say, fortified infant formula, and also giving the recommended NHS vitamin drops – could the baby get too much?

Here is a comparison for a baby of 6 months (Table 2.7):

Table 2.7   Overdosing?

	Average daily intake from				DHSS recommended intake at 6 months
	Vitamin drops	600ml formula	40g weaning food	Total	
Vitamin A:	200ug	480ug	280ug	960ug	450ug
Vitamin C:	20mg	48mg	20mg	88mg	20mg
Vitamin D:	7ug	7ug	6ug	20ug	8ug
Iron:		3mg	14mg	17mg	6mg
Calcium:		510mg	400mg	910mg	600mg

Sources   Product labels; DHSS RDAs.

There seems to be an excess of vitamins – as much as 400 per cent of the recommended levels. This may not be a hazard in the case of Vitamin C, as our bodies simply excrete the excess. For Vitamin A, it is now thought there are several types of this vitamin, and it is possible that an excess of one sort could block the uptake of other, also valuable, sorts – we simply do not know.

For Vitamin D there are reports that some individuals can suffer from excess levels, especially if they are also getting excess calcium – which can, in rare cases, lead to hypercalcaemia, with the risk of kidney damage. There may also be a link between excess Vitamin D and heart disease. One researcher has suggested that, with Vitamin D-fortified breakfast cereal, margarine, follow-up milk and the recommended vitamin drops from the clinic, a baby may go way above safe limits. In Canada, commercial fortification of food is now strictly regulated.

High levels of iron – the fortified iron used in infant formula – have been associated with impairment of the ability to absorb essential copper. And, as we mentioned, high levels of calcium can, in rare cases, lead to hypercalcaemia.

The problem is that we just don't know what effects such high doses might have, especially if there are insufficient quantities of other nutrients. It is only recently that such levels of these pure, synthetic forms of nutrients have been offered to babies. They are the experimental generation – on them we shall evaluate the good or bad effects of these foods.

READY-TO-EAT DINNERS

Take a look at the list of ingredients (Fig. 2.7). For many products the first thing you will find is *water*. If water is first on the list then it means that there is more water in the product than any other single item. Here are two examples:

Ingredients: WATER, LOW FAT YOGHURT, RASPBERRIES, SUGAR, MODIFIED CORNFLOUR, CHERRIES, MAIZE OIL, VITAMIN C.

Approximate composition per 100g

ENERGY 263kj/62kcal	CARBOHYDRATE 14.1g
PROTEIN 1.3g	FAT 0.4g

Contains not less than 25mg Vitamin C per 100g

INGREDIENTS: WATER, EGGS, BACON, RICE
DRIED SKIMMED MILK, MODIFIED CORNFLOUR, SOYA FLOUR
VEGETABLE OIL, CORNFLOUR, VITAMIN B1

	FAT	PROTEIN	CARBOHYDRATE	ENERGY
		NUTRITIONAL ANALYSIS OF PRODUCT		
Per can	3.8g	4.5g	7.9g	340 kj (82 kcal)
Per 100g	3.0g	3.5g	6.2g	270 kj (64 kcal)

Figure 2.7

If you make these foods yourself from a cookery book then you are unlikely to find that water is the largest ingredient in the recipe. So what is going on?

TRADE TACTICS – SELL 'EM WATER

Obviously the product with water at the top, or near the top of its ingredient list is fairly dilute, and probably more dilute than we would make it at home. More water is present than we would think of adding. Are we being sold water instead of food? The manufacturers would say that water is necessary to help 'improve the flowing qualities' and 'create a uniform consistency' ensuring every item is the same. But they would say that, wouldn't they?

If we open the tin or jar does the water pour out? It does not. That wouldn't do at all – we would see too soon how we were getting a thin sauce instead of a ˜ thick purée. How do the manufacturers stop the water from looking like water? They use thickening agents: the cheap and readily available starches and gums – cornflour, modified cornflour, soya flour, wheat flour, potato flour, plain starch and modified starch.

These starches added to thicken the purée are usually highly refined with very little nutrient value of their own. The poor nutritional value is probably of little importance, because it only takes a little of the stuff to thicken a lot of watery sauce. Just like the cornflour or farina we use at home, a couple of spoonfuls can thicken a pint or more.

Just *how much* thickened water is being put in these products is very difficult to establish. Ingredients lists like these (Fig. 2.8) list several different types of thickener:

INGREDIENTS:

Water, Cheese, Onions,
Thickener (Modified Cornflour), Tomato
Purée, Macaroni, Soya Protein, Full Cream
Milk Powder.

INGREDIENTS: WATER, PORK, POTATOES, CARROTS, FLOUR
TOMATO PUREE, PEARL BARLEY, GELATINE, MODIFIED
CORNFLOUR, HYDROLYSED VEGETABLE PROTEIN
IRON SULPHATE (iron 2mg/100g), HERBS

NUTRITIONAL ANALYSIS OF PRODUCT

	FAT	PROTEIN	CARBOHYDRATE	ENERGY
Per can	4.5g	4.5g	11.4g	424 kj (101 kcal)
Per 100g	3.5g	3.5g	8.9g	331 kj (79 kcal)

Figure 2.8

In the last of these there are – if you include the vegetable thickeners, like potatoes, tomato purée, etc. – some seven different thickening agents.

The impression is that they have put a lot of water in these products, but the labels do not tell us. We have no rights, under present labelling laws, to know how much of anything there is in these products. As nutritionist Caroline Walker has pointed out, we know how much cotton is in our baby's socks because the label gives the details, but we don't have the same details about what goes in our baby's mouth.

> How much unnecessary thickener is put into baby foods? One US company, Beech Nut, proposed in 1985 that it was considering reformulating its products, without the added starches, natural or modified. The company admitted that if they were to make this change some of their products would have as much as *25 per cent more vegetables and up to 50 per cent more meat* than they had before. It would be interesting to see similar proposals, and similar admissions, from baby food manufacturers in Britain.

Another area of concern, which is made all the worse by our present labelling regulations, is the nature and quality of the meat being used in the meat-containing products. In 1986, all meat products sold to the public were supposed to say on the label how much meat there was inside them. The manufacturers also had to ensure that a certain percentage of this meat (usually 65 per cent) was lean meat. (We look in more detail at meat products and some tricks of the meat trade in a later section.)

For reasons we have not been able to fathom, the baby food companies have not had to comply with these labelling regulations. They can put as much or as little meat in the jar as they like, and still put the meat as a big feature on the front. Look hard at the label and you still won't know the meat content, you won't know the lean meat, and you won't know what parts of the animal have been included, or even if there are other animals' meat besides the ones indicated (e.g. there can be pork meat or fat in products called 'Beef').

It might be that we are getting a good bargain. We could be

getting top-quality cuts of lean meat, put into the product in generous proportions. Or we could be getting chicken skin, pork rind, headmeat, tailmeat, bowels or feet – as food manufacturers may use in other products. We simply do not know and we have no right to be told.

One form of meat that some manufacturers use now is called Mechanically Recovered Meat (MRM). After an animal carcass has had the meat removed there are still a few shreds of meat, and sinew, gristle and other connective tissues attached to the bones, so these bones are put through a high pressure tumbler or scraper to strip off these remaining pieces. This produces a 'slurry' or paste of small particles of 'meat' which may be thickened, coloured or flavoured and put into various meat products like sausages and pies. The nutritional value is not considered to be as good as lean meat, and there are some questions about its potential to harbour bacteria.

One danger of this MRM is that bits of bone may get squeezed or chipped off, and that the bone gets mixed into the meat product. If the bone particles are very small, then it might be argued that this is just a nutritious source of extra calcium. But if the bits are larger then there could just be a hazard – especially for small, young throats.

We have no evidence that MRM *is* being used for baby products. Nor do we have evidence that it is not. The labels do not say and the companies are unlikely to volunteer the details. But the question of MRM was raised in the case of Heinz's rapid withdrawal of 300,000 tins of Baby Strained Beef and Oxtail Dinner in 1986, following the discovery of 'small pieces of bone, resembling grains of rice' in the product. We are not saying that MRM was being used in that product, only that it might have been – we do not know. And under the present regulations we have no right to find out.

A baby may not care if there is not much meat in the dinner, or indeed not much flavour generally. But although the baby may be indifferent, the person feeding the baby may find the taste to be very bland, and might suspect that the quality was poor. They might suspect that there was too much water, or too little meat, or too few vegetables ... If the adult thinks that the meals taste too bland then they might start wondering if the product was actually much good and had anything useful in it. Meat and vegetables made at home would not taste so weak. So, the adult wonders, is there anything nutritious in this stuff? Maybe not.

To get around the problem of a 'weak' taste for adults manufacturers used to rely on adding a pinch of salt and even some monosodium glutamate. But now monosodium glutamate (a flavour enhancer) has been banned from baby foods, and the DHSS has been saying for several years that no salt should be added (though it is still legal to do so). Putting 'No added salt' and 'No flavour enhancer' on the label is a bonus – but how will the taste get topped up?

Increasingly manufacturers have turned to alternatives. Herbs and spices are one solution. There may be no problem from a

INGREDIENTS:

Water, Beef, Potatoes, Tomatoes,
Onions, Thickener (Modified Cornflour),
Peas, Soya Protein, Hydrolysed
Vegetable Protein.

Ingredients: WATER, BACON, TOMATOES,
POTATOES, MODIFIED CORNFLOUR, EGG, SOYA
PROTEIN, ONIONS HYDROLYSED VEGETABLE
PROTEIN.

Approximate composition per 100g
ENERGY   222kj/53kcalCARBOHYDRATE   4.6g
PROTEIN   3.5gFAT   2.4g

Figure 2.9

dietary point of view, but their presence may indicate that the product is otherwise bland. Manufacturers are also using various proteins such as those extracted from meat and from yeast, including *hydrolysed vegetable protein* (HVP). These act as flavour boosters (Fig. 2.9). Although they are not termed flavour enhancers by the regulating authority (the Ministry of Agriculture, Fisheries and Food) their role is still to add a flavour kick to the food. HVP has a savoury flavour and can enhance the 'meatiness' of the product. It has compounds related to the glutamates, as it is regarded by some researchers as a possible hazard (see Chapter 4, Reading the Small Print). As with the herbs and spices, its presence may well indicate a product that would otherwise taste thin and bland.

In 1986, Heinz declared in America that it would be removing all pesticide residues from their baby products, listing twelve chemicals which were in current use on farms. All crops would be examined for pesticides before being accepted.

Some of the same chemicals are used in farms in Europe, but Heinz has not announced a ban on their presence in baby food here.

Milupa, on the other hand, claims that all its ingredients are examined for pesticides, and the meats are also examined for hormone levels.

British food regulations are of little help here. Manufacturers are not obliged to test for these residues, and they don't have to say whether they have tested or not. Only consumer pressure will force them to declare what they are doing.

In summary, we can deduce certain things by looking carefully at the jars and packets. We can see how starches can replace nutritious foods, and can be used to thicken and bulk out a poor product. We can see if the manufacturers think extra flavour boosters are needed. But we cannot tell how important and relevant these things may be because the details are not shown: there is no indication of how much extra water is present, or how much carrot, potato or chicken might be there. We do not know enough about the meat, because the labels say very little. We do not know these things and under present regulations we have no right to know.

TEETHING RUSKS OR TEETHING RISKS

The baby's gums are sore and its teeth are starting to come through. Something nice to massage the gums might help – but for the tooth's sake it had better not be sugar ... surely?

Dried bread, crusts and toast make perfectly adequate teething rusks. In fact they are more adequate compared with the rusks sold in the chemists and supermarkets. Commercial rusks are more like regular sweet biscuits. Table 2.8 shows the sugar content of commercial rusks, compared with bread and dough-nuts.

Not only are these rusks sold as suitable for babies to chew on at the time their teeth are coming through, but they are also sold

Table 2.8   Weaning onto sweet snacks

Brands	Per cent sugars in each biscuit	Cost per ounce
Farley, original	31	9p–15p
Farley, low	23.5	9p–15p
Farex Fingers	28	8p
Cow & Gate, liga	16	12p
Milupa Fruit Rusks	19.5	15p
Boots, regular	26	7p
Boots Apricot, low	19	8p
Doughnut	15	5p
Bread	2	3p
Bikkipegs	0	41p

Sources   Product labels; McCance and Widdowson, *The Composition of Foods*.

as suitable for the baby's first solid food. 'Safe, gentle and nourishing' promises one 'low sugar' (23.5 per cent sugars) rusk. 'When it is time to start weaning ... crush a small piece of rusk in a bowl with the back of a spoon.' Add milk or water and you have ' ... an ideal food for your baby'.

Furthermore, one manufacturer declared that the sugar was essential in the rusk, precisely because the rusks were used as weaning foods. Writing to the Maternity Alliance about their policies on adding sugar to baby foods, Cow & Gate (who make liga rusks) declared that the sugar in their rusks was 'necessary in this type of product if it is intended to break down in breastmilk, babymilk or water and hence provide a source of nutrients in the baby's diet'.

The same company produces glossy leaflets stating, quite correctly: 'it is not recommended that babies are fed foods which are highly seasoned or flavoured particularly with added salt or sugar ... Sugar is used to sweeten the flavour of foods and, although a useful energy source, provides no further food value.' And 'That is why Cow & Gate have developed a rusk with such a low sugar content.'

Nowhere in their leaflets do Cow & Gate, who call themselves 'The Babyfeeding Specialists', list the sugar levels of their products (though they do give helpful hints on how to stop breast-feeding and start bottle-feeding, and they also suggest that cow's milk should be boiled before giving to a baby – something most dieticians say is unnecessary and destroys valuable vitamins in the milk).

In the end, we are left with some ambiguity. The rusks are described by the company as 'Perfect for weaning and teething', yet they produce a rusk with more sugar than doughnuts. They state that sugar is undesirable in baby foods, but then they add it to a teething rusk in order that the teething rusk can also be sold as a baby's first solid weaning food. All very confusing.

CALL ME Al

There are strict laws about some contaminating metals in our food. Tinned foods have rigid limits on the quantity of lead permissible. Other metals, especially 'heavy' metals which can be harmful, have regulations and recommendations concerning their presence in food. But not aluminium. Aluminium is a relatively 'recent' metal in the sense that few objects were manufactured from aluminium before the beginning of this century. Now it is one of the commonest metals in the household – especially in the kitchen. But should we be eating it?

We know that kidney patients can suffer irreversible brain damage if too much aluminium accumulates in their blood. We know that babies can absorb much more metal from the same proportional intake compared with adults, and their retention of aluminium in the brain will be higher. We know that premature babies are at special risk because their kidneys have not developed their full functions. Aluminium in the diet is also thought to play a part in children's learning problems, and in the development of the illness, Alzheimer's disease, a form of senile dementia.

There are no 'acceptable levels' of aluminium recommended by the government. The European Community has set an upper limit of 200 micrograms per litre of water (ug/1). The DHSS recommends that kidney patients should not be given more then 30 micrograms per litre (ug/1). Tap water in some areas can be high in aluminium – up to 300 ug/1, and over 200 ug/1 in many areas in England and Wales.

There are no limits to the aluminium content of baby feeds. It would seem a sensible precaution, given the levels in some water supplies, and the possible contamination from cooking implements, that the levels of aluminium in commercial baby products should be as low as possible. Yet a recent survey by Warwickshire County Council Trading Standards Department found aluminium to be present in baby foods, sometimes in quite large quantities. They used water containing only 35 ug/1 in making up some of the baby foods listed below, but found that far higher levels were already present in the food:

Table 2.9   Aluminium in baby foods

Infant formula	as much as 840 ug/1
Baby drinks	330 ug/1
Soya drink	720 ug/1
Cauliflower cheese dinner	600 ug/1
Beef stew and vegetables	3100 ug/1
Savoury chicken and rice	3700 ug/1

Source   Warwick County Council Trading Standards Dept.

The amounts actually involved may not be dangerous. We do not know. Only future generations can tell us.

MAIN MENUS FOR LIFE

By the age of 9 months to a year, a baby will start to have the food that the rest of the family eats. This is the time when the habits of a lifetime will start to be formed. The sorts of food being eaten at this age will have a long-term influence on their growth and development and their future health prospects.

Very few research studies have looked closely at the sort of diets being eaten by young children after they stop eating the proprietary weaning foods and start eating the sorts of food eaten by their brothers and sisters. The main study available on what is happening at present is one looking at children under the age of 2 years, in a low-income area in West Glamorgan. The proportions of children falling well below the nutritional levels recommended by the DHSS was large for many of the key nutrients needed by children. When the researchers looked at how the children's diet changed as they were weaned onto solid foods and onto foods eaten by the rest of the family they found a worsening of the overall nutritional quality as the children got older. The better, earlier nutrition was, they believed, due in part to the breast-milk, formula milk and the fortification in the weaning foods. Even the period when they were moving towards weaning foods saw a decline in nutritional quality, especially in the nutrients that are less often fortified in commercial weaning food brands – such as magnesium and Vitamin E. And as they started eating regular food their nutrient intake across the spectrum of essential nutrients dropped to very low levels.

What sort of food are children eating once they leave behind the specially prepared weaning foods? As we saw earlier in this book, the trends nationally are away from fresh foods and towards more processed foods – and just these sorts of foods are promoted by the manufacturers directly at younger children. Take breakfast cereals. The very first thing we eat in the morning has seen just this transformation – gone are the plain porridge oats, and in their place are bright new wonder-food breakfast cereals, many of which are marketed for younger children.

YOUR STARTER FOR SIX – BREAKFAST CEREALS

More than six out of every ten children now begin their day with a
bowlful of ready-to-eat packet breakfast cereal. Breakfast cereals
have come to replace the old porridge oats breakfast, and now
dominate our morning tables. We buy as a nation around 20
million packets of ready-to-eat breakfast cereals each week, eating
more per person than any other country in the world.

Nutritional analyses of processed breakfast cereals found
that many of the vitamins present in the original grains had
been largely destroyed by the processing techniques used to
turn them into the puffed, crunchy, flaky products we now
buy. Indeed, some of these ready-to-eat cereals appeared to be
so low in nutrients that it was rumoured that experimental
animals lived longer if they ate the packet rather than the
cereals inside.

As a result of the concern over the poor nutritional value
manufacturers started to fortify their products. It is the same
story we have met before: refined processed foods which are so
lacking in nutrients that they have to have vitamin pills added to
make them worth eating.

Cereal foods are recommended by dietitians as they can be a
valuable source of nutrients and dietary fibre. Wholegrain
varieties of breakfast cereal contain all the nutrients one can
expect from cereal foods, although some may have been lost
during processing. Non-wholegrain cereals can be very low
on natural nutrients and will probably have some added
back in as fortification. Some will also have added pure bran,
and some will be largely made of bran with some salt and
sugar to make it palatable. Adding extra bran to a cereal food
may prevent some essential nutrients from being well
absorbed, and so might not be of long-term benefit. The
digestive system is designed to work best with a variety of
types of fibre (from fruit, vegetables and pulses as well as
cereals) eaten in their 'wholefood' forms. We simply do not
know whether pure refined bran is an adequate substitute
for dietary fibre from wholegrain sources, and there is some
evidence that it might not be.

Besides the powdered vitamin pills, and perhaps the added bran, many breakfast cereal products are sprinkled with iron. In many cases, this isn't iron in the form you might find it in meat and liver, spinach or dried fruit. It is iron in the form you find it in cars, ships and railways – plain iron like nuts and bolts. A letter in the medical journal, *The Lancet*, claimed that much of this iron came as a by-product of the scrap car industry. The body can't use this form of iron very easily, and so about ten times as much as we need is put into the cereals, just to ensure that a bit of it will be absorbed, and the manufacturers can truly claim that they have added iron to our diets. This iron powder may be the least of our worries, though.

TRADE TACTICS – A SWEET BY ANY OTHER NAME

The top cereals from the advertisers point of view are the ones promoted in children's prime-time television. Both the advertising and the images presented on the packet, along with the special offers and free gifts, identify these cereals as being aimed particularly at younger children.

There is one thing that stands out about these highly promoted and advertised breakfast cereals. Compared with the rest of the cereals on the shop shelves, they are all high in sugar. In fact the top two have more sugar, weight for weight, than many confectionary products, like fruit gums or Bounty bars (Table 2.10):

Table 2.10   Breakfast cereal – or candy?

Product	Sugars as % of weight
Bounty bar	54
Fruit gums	43
Products aimed at younger children	
Sugar Puffs	57
Frosties	43
Ricicles	40
Coco Pops	38
Honey Smacks	39
Start	32
Other brand leaders	
Corn flakes	7

Table 2.10 *continued*

Puffed Wheat	0
Rice Crispies	11
Shredded Wheat	1
Weetabix	6

Products with a 'health' image

All Bran	15
Bran Buds	26
Tropical Fruit Alpen	22
Fruit 'n' Fibre	27
Farmhouse Bran	23
Harvest Crunch	18
Special K	18
Sultana Bran	33

Source McCance and Widdowson, *The Composition of Foods* (3rd Supplement).

THE SUGAR JAG

The sugar in processed foods like breakfast cereals will be quickly digested and quickly burnt – especially if not much protein, fat or dietary fibre has been eaten at the same time. The blood sugar levels in the body will rise rapidly and then may fall as the sugar gets converted by insulin. This dip in blood sugar levels could make a child feel lethargic and tired.

The blood sugar boost followed by a dip is called a sugar 'jag' and can have the effect of making the person feel hungry again. A mid-morning snack is wanted – perhaps a sweet drink and a biscuit. More sugar, another blood sugar boost and then another dip, and the sugar jag is repeated.

We simply do not know what the long-term effects of eating this way may have on our physiology. There may be immediately noticeable changes of mood and periods of high activity followed by periods of lethargy. In the long term these rushes of sugar may have no effect or they may provoke problems in the body's ability to handle sugar. We do not know. But it is a sad fact that the numbers of adults suffering and dying from diabetes has risen remarkably in the last ten to twenty years, and in Professor Yudkin's recently reissued *Pure, White and Deadly*, diabetes along with several other diseases (caries, myopia, dermatitis, dyspepsia, gout, cancer and heart disease) is considered to be associated with sugar consumption over long periods.

Even if we try to find a healthy alternative we may have a problem. Muesli bars and their look-alike relatives (Fig. 2.10) now take up considerable space on the shop shelves – but are they any better for us? In many cases the answer is no – they will be loaded with calories, fats and teeth-rotting sugars. Look carefully at the ingredient listings of these 'healthy' alternative snacks:

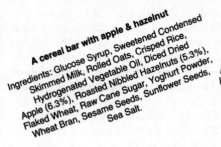

A cereal bar with apple & hazelnut

Ingredients: Glucose Syrup, Sweetened Condensed Skimmed Milk, Rolled Oats, Crisped Rice, Hydrogenated Vegetable Oil, Diced Dried Apple (6.3%), Roasted Nibbled Hazelnuts (5.3%), Flaked Wheat, Raw Cane Sugar, Yoghurt Powder, Wheat Bran, Sesame Seeds, Sunflower Seeds, Sea Salt.

Ingredients: Rolled Oats, Raw Sugar, Soya Oil, Honey (6%), Almonds (6%), Hazelnuts, Bran, Wheatgerm, Sesame Seeds, Sunflower Seeds, Molasses, Sea Salt, Lecithin, Pure Vanilla and Almond Extract.

Ingredients:
Rolled Oats, Glucose Syrup,
Corn Syrup Solids, Whole
Rolled Wheat, Mixed Nuts
(9%), (Peanuts, Almonds,
Hazelnuts), Raisins (8.5%),
Crisp Rice, Hydrogenated
Vegetable Oil, Honey,
Sunflower Seeds, Glycerol,
Brown Sugar, Dried Skimmed
Milk, Raisin Juice, Sorbitol,
Salt, Dried Unsweetened
Coconut, Flavouring,
Antioxidant E320.

Figure 2.10

But by giving these 'health' bars we may at least feel that we are not giving any suspected additives, and that we might be giving some useful nutrients, buried somewhere in the bar. And to an extent we would be right, because elsewhere in the food industry they have dreamed up a whole new technology providing snacks that are virtually empty of all nutrition, being mostly calories, salt and additives – extruded and moulded snack pellets.

EXTRUDED SNACK PELLETS

The last ten years has seen the arrival of an enormous variety of
savoury snacks in brightly coloured bags. These are called, in the
trade, 'bag snacks' and include the familiar crisps and salted nuts
along with the newer forms of processed, puffed-up crunchy
wonder food. These last sorts are the ones which are arriving in
big numbers, and are worth over quarter of a billion pounds in
sales for the manufacturers.

Most of the products consist of a puffed corn starch or potato
starch base, extruded or moulded and fried, and then coated with
extra flavourings and flavour enhancers to make the most of what is
there. In most cases the products are 'extruded snack pellets', a
process whereby dehydrated pellets of starch, which can be easily
transported in bulk and which last for years, are reconstituted into a
paste, and the paste is pushed at high pressure through a small,
shaped hole. As the paste squeezes through it gets very hot and puffs
out, so creating whatever shape the machine's designer has chosen.

What we get nutritionally is highly processed starch, plus whatever fats, sugars, salt, flavourings and other ingredients manufacturers want to put in the paste, in the frying oils or sprinkle onto the
extruded product afterwards. The result is virtually the same
product in a whole range of different forms – and the story is one of
low-nutrient calories. Most of the goodness has been destroyed.
Even if extra vitamins are added into the paste during production
they will be destroyed. Here are some figures from recent research
into vitamin losses during the extrusion process (Table 2.11).

Table 2.11   Loss of vitamins in extrusion

Vitamins	% loss in extrusion
Vitamin A	up to 88%
Vitamin B1	up to 62%
Vitamin B2	up to 40%
Vitamin B6	up to 44%
Vitamin B12	up to 40%
Niacin	up to 40%
Folic acid	up to 65%
Vitamin C	up to 87%
Vitamin E	up to 86%

Source   Colm O'Connor (ed.), *Extrusion Technology for the Food
Industry*, Elsevier, 1987.

ADDITIVES IN SNACKS

One of the few success stories where we consumers may feel we can congratulate ourselves is the attack we have made on additives in bag snacks and soft drinks. The years of complaining about the additives in crisps and orange squash have had some effect. But the effect is perhaps less than the publicity the manufacturers have made, and the front of the packets seem to imply. It is still difficult to get low-fat varieties of crisps, and only one manufacturer (Smiths) allows us to choose how much salt we want.

Gone from some bag snacks	*But still there in others*
Colours: Azo dyes	Colours: Caramel, Annatto
Flavour enhancers	Flavour enhancers
Antioxidants: BHA, BHT	Antioxidants: BHA, BHT

And of course still there in all of them is the fat, salt, and undisclosed flavouring agents. (For more details on these additives see Chapter 4.)

The same is true for soft drinks like squashes, barley waters, and fruit drinks. Some of the old horrors have been ousted from some ingredient lists, but there is still some distance to go:

Gone from some squash bottles	*But still there in others*
Colours: Azo dyes	Colours: Annatto, Beta-carotene
Preservatives: Benzoates	Preservatives: Sulphites, Benzoates
Flavourings	Flavourings

And of course there is still the sugar. (For more details on these additives see Chapter 4.)

TRADE TACTICS – THE VANISHING ORANGE

It is fairly easy to take orange juice and add sugar and water and still sell it as having all the goodness of oranges in it. The potential for abusing orange juice products has led to standards being set by the Ministry of Agriculture, Fisheries and Food (MAFF) defining the amount of juice that must be present in a squash. The amount is not very high. Concentrated squashes should contain a minimum 25 per cent of fruit juice (this means around 5 per cent after normal dilution). If juice is not used, but instead a pulp of minced fruit is used, then the product is not a squash but a drink. Minced fruit is called 'comminuted' and means that the whole fruit – pith, skin and flesh – will be there.

For all its faults, the standards offered some protection from being sold rubbish. Now, however, we are heading for a change in the standards. As we go to press, there are proposals being drafted by MAFF to abolish these requirements and leave it up to the customers to read the label carefully if they want to know if there is any fruit in the bottle. The idea is that there will be no minimum level of fruit, only a declaration somewhere on the label saying what is actually in the pack.

The same logic, part of what the Ministry calls 'lifting the burden' from manufacturers, was recently applied to meat and fish products – the standards were replaced by label declarations – and the effect was an alarming drop in the average levels of meat and fish present in these products. Trading Standards Officers all over the country reported declining amounts of meat in meat products. The same may well happen in the case of fruit squashes and fruit drinks. They may not be much good for us now, but the chances are that they will get no better in the near future. The juice will vanish into the small print.

Here is another confusing labelling law. If the packet says *orange flavoured drink* then there will be only a very little fruit inside, far less than the 25 per cent which has been required for *orange drink* or *orange squash* concentrates.

And if the pack says *orange flavour drink* then there will probably be nothing at all inside that came from the fruit of an orange, though there may be a chemical flavouring agent to give an 'orange' taste, and a colouring to give an 'orange' colour (Fig. 2.11).

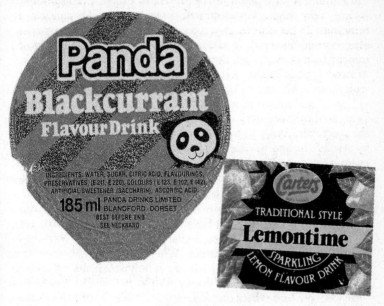

Figure 2.11

FISHY TALES

What do young children like to eat at dinner time? What does a parent know will be accepted when presented on a plate? The answer often comes back: fish fingers, sausages, and burgers.

Let us take a close look at fish fingers. Once upon a time they consisted of plain fish, coated in a thin layer of breadcrumbs. That was several years ago. Gradually manufacturers started to rival each other in the 'golden' colour of the breadcrumbs, to make them look freshly fried, and in came the notorious colouring agents like tartrazine and sunset yellow.

But recently our concerns about these additives have led the manufacturers to fall over themselves in seeing how quickly they could make fish fingers attractive without these dyes. Now we find the supermarket freezers stuffed with fish fingers that boast their lack of artificial colouring – but they are still coloured! The new dyes are ones which can be found in various species of plant, and so the manufacturers have given themselves a licence to call these 'natural' colourings, but the colourings are by no means a natural part of the breadcrumbs. (Furthermore, these additives may not be as thoroughly tested as the old-fashioned, artificial additives – for more on additives see Chapter 5.)

We may feel that we have had a victory of sorts, because at least the azo dyes have gone. But while all this fuss about the breadcrumb colourings was going on, manufacturers have been quietly doing something else to the fish fingers which we have not noticed. They have been taking out the fish.

Those unsung heroes of our time – the local authority food inspectors (public analysts, environmental health officers and trading standards officers) – have been taking a look inside the breadcrumbs to see what was happening to the fishy bit itself – and what they found alarmed them (Table 2.12). Where once there was a whole piece of fillet fish they found, in many cases, bits of chewed up fish mince, reshaped and re-formed into single strips of look-alike solid pieces. Where once the fish was plain fish, the flesh was now being soaked in polyphosphate solution to absorb water. More water means weight-for-weight less fish in each finger. And where once there was a large bit of fish in a thin coat of crumb, now there was a much smaller bit in a thicker coat.

Table 2.12   Fish in a fish finger

1962:	78%	average
	68%	worst
1968:	65%	average
	52%	worst
1976:	58%	average
	50%	worst
1983:	57%	average
	33%	worst

Source   Institute of Trading Standards Administration.

The total effect was a decline in the quality of fish fingers, with an average loss of over a quarter of the original fish from a typical product, and a loss of more than half the fish in the worst examples.

With some products offering about one-third of their weight in fish, and costing 6 pence or even 8 pence each, the real cost of the fish is around £2.80p–£3.60p for a pound weight – a pound of what may be re-formed fish mince. A careful shopper could buy off-cuts of smoked salmon for that sort of money, or at least some good quality (and far more nutritious) prime cod fillets

SAUSAGES AND BURGERS – HUNT THE MEAT

One of the fishy tricks in fish fingers is also used with sausages. Get the meat to soak up water and you can sell the water for the price of the meat. Look carefully at the list of ingredients (Fig. 2.12) and see if there is a liberal sprinkling of polyphosphates (or their 'E' numbers: E450a, E450b or E450c).

MINIMUM 65% MEAT

INGREDIENTS:
Pork, Water, Rusk, Starch, Salt,
Caseinates, Sodium Polyphosphate, Sugar
Preservative (E223), Flavourings, Wheat
flour, Autolysed Yeast, Antioxidants (E304,
307), Spices, Colour (E128).

KEEP REFRIGERATED

MINIMUM 65% MEAT

INGREDIENTS
PORK, WATER, RUSKS, STARCH, SALT, SODIUM POLYPHOSPHATES,
SPICES, PRESERVATIVE (E221), ANTIOXIDANT (E301).
0245 Produced in the U.K. for Tesco stores LTd, Cheshunt, Herts. © Tesco 1986.

INGREDIENTS: PORK, WATER, RUSK, BEEF, STARCH, SALT, INGREDIENTS LESS THAN 1%: SOYA PROTEIN
CONCENTRATE, SPICES, TRIPHOSPHATES, ANTIOXIDANTS (VITAMINS C AND E), HERBS, PRESERVATIVE
E223 COLOUR 128. MINIMUM 51% MEAT, INGREDIENTS CONTAINED AT LESS THAN 1% INCLUDE:
TRIPHOSPHATES – TO KEEP PRODUCT TEXTURE, ANTIOXIDANTS – TO PREVENT DISCOLOURATION.

Figure 2.12

These are the favourite water-absorbers used by the meat companies to boost the weight of the meat. Then there are emulsifiers.

These help bind fat and water together, which is fine if you want a smooth milk shake, or mayonnaise or even a non-drip paint. But they are not fine when you expect lean meat. The manufacturers will tell you that these tricks all give their products a 'better bite' or 'improved mouth feel' or even 'enhanced organoleptic qualities' which means the same. But from the consumer's point of view they all add up to one thing: these additives help to bolster the texture of the coloured, fatty paste, with its thickeners of rusk and soya flour, which has the nerve to claim the historical traditions of the British sausage.

Incidentally, the actual lean meat in a standard beef sausage is less than you might think. A regular-sized sausage (at eight for one pound weight) can, under the 1984 regulations, have *less than three teaspoons* of lean meat in it. Not, you might feel, a generous amount for a growing child. What is more, not all of the meat in a beef sausage needs to be beef, but can include pork, chicken, turkey or other animal meats – even if the label says 'beef sausages'.

A similar story can be told for burgers. Though we cannot claim a British tradition for burgers, we can claim some special ways of impoverishing the product. The original 'flat meatball' was plain ground beef with a few herbs. If it was too fatty it fell apart while cooking, so only lean beef was used. But what do we have now? Here are the ingredients from some retail burgers (Fig. 2.13):

Ingredients:

Water, Pork, Other Meat, Tomato, Starch,
Onion, Wheat Flour, Salt, Yeast Extract,
Flavouring, Sodium Caseinate, Polyphosphate
E450(C), Spices
Minimum, 35% Meat

INGREDIENTS

Beef (minimum 80%), Fresh Onion,
Rusk, Soya, Protein, Beef & Onion
Seasoning, Salt, Spices, Flavour
Enhancer (621), Preservative (E223),
Produce of the United Kingdom

INGREDIENTS

Beef, onion, rusk, salt, soya flour
concentrate, hydrolysed vegetable,
protein, preservative (E223), sugar,
wheatflour, flavour enhancers
(6231,635), onion powder, spices,
colour (128).

Minimum meat content 80%

Figure 2.13

As with the sausages, the meat content is far from 100 per cent, and even the declared meat content can be up to one-third pure fat, with only two-thirds lean meat. Just like sausages, there are the polyphosphates to hold extra water, and there are the colourings and the bulking rusks and flours. And the meat may not be pure beef but can be other animals, and it can be from various bits of the body such as tailmeat, headmeat, feet, skin, sinew and mechanically recovered meat (just as we described in the section on ready-to-eat baby foods).

What is in a name? A *100% beef burger* can have added water (up to 15%) and added fat (up to 35%). An *economy burger* can be 40% non-meat, and even the parts that are meat can be one-third pure fat.

A *beefburger* need not be pure beef, but can have up to 20% other animals' meat in it (e.g. pig, chicken, turkey, pork rind or lard). So an *economy beef burger* could be, quite legally, 40% pure pig fat.

Obviously this sort of food adulteration matters a lot to people who want to avoid certain meats or meats from certain animals for cultural reasons. A buyer cannot tell by looking at the label whether the product might contain, for example, pork or pig fat (lard). Under present regulations the label does not have to give this detail, and the buyer has no right to know.

We can ask whether this matters from a nutritional point of view. Will our children still get what they need? In Table 2.13 there is a comparison, showing the nutrients you get if you stoke yourself up on 100 calories of stewing steak compared with 100 calories of a typical burger.

As can be seen, the nutrient levels per 100 calories of a burger can be substantially lower than they are in fairly cheap beef (stewing steak).

FAST FOOD AND TAKE-AWAYS

Eating food from take-away and fast food restaurants is often an easy and convenient means of getting oneself or one's child fed. It

Table 2.13   Nutrients in 100 calories-worth of meat

	Stewing steak	Beefburger
Protein	14g	8g
Iron	1.3mg	1.2mg
Vitamin B1	13ug	8ug
Vitamin B2	143ug	87ug
Vitamin B6	130ug	76ug
Vitamin B12	0.9ug	0.8ug
Niacin	4.6mg	3.0mg

Source   McCance and Widdowson, *The Composition of Foods*.

offers a major advantage over home cooking, in that each person can choose from the menu what they wish to have. Many an argument with a tired and hungry child has been saved by a trip to the take-away. But is take-away food really junk? Is there really such a choice, and more importantly, is it possible to get a balanced and healthy meal?

The London Food Commission has looked in some detail at the content of commercial fast foods – asking what the nutritional values of these meals are and also what other ingredients might be present which the eater does not expect. Very few ingredients lists are available to a casual eater, and the packages are not on display, so there is no easy way to find out what actually goes into this food. In the LFC survey we found good and bad products, some well worth eating and others of less useful nutritional quality, and some with various additives which suggested poor quality indeed – in other words, a range of foods much like the range available from other sections of the food industry, some good, some bad and some indifferent.

In Table 2.14 is a summary of what the LFC found.

TRADE TACTICS – THE HI-TECH FIX

Imagine cakes, cream buns, confectionery ... all calorie-free! Imagine hot dogs and hamburgers, milk shakes and french fries ... all calorie-free! Then talk to the biochemists and find that all this and more besides may soon be possible.

The future is nearly here. We already have artificial sweeteners, but soon we can expect rejigged sugar molecules with trade names like *sucralose* which are just like sugar but cannot be digested. We already have low-fat spreads, but soon we can expect chemically rejigged foods with trade names like *olestra* which can be cooked like fat but cannot be digested. And we already have starch-reduced crispbreads, but soon we can expect *fluffy cellulose* which can be cooked like starch but which cannot be digested.

We can soon have these 100 per cent calorie-free sugars, fats and starches, spun and woven into any textures and mixtures we want – and even sprinkled with powdered vitamins to keep us alive. All this comes courtesy of your local chemical industry. No one quite knows what problems these 'foods' might lead to in the human population. But what the heck – we will find out soon enough! At least, our children will ...

Table 2.14 A fast look at fast foods

Meal item	Good points	Bad points	Needed to balance	NOTE!
Fish and chips	Protein, calcium, Vitamins B6, B12	High fat, many other vitamins low	Fresh veg and fruit, lean meat, wholegrains	Tartrazine in batter
Fried chicken and chips	Protein, Vitamins B3, B6	High fat, many other vitamins low	Fruit and vegetables, fish, wholegrains	Monosodium glutamate in coating
Doner kebab with salad	Protein, zinc, some vitamins	High fat, a few vitamins low	More salad, fruit and wholegrains, pulses	Meat fatty, otherwise good
Shish kebab with salad	Protein, calcium, iron, zinc, some vitamins	A few vitamins low	Vegetables, pulses	Good, and try with humus & extra salad
Sweet & sour chicken and egg fried rice	Protein, iron, calcium	High fat, a few vitamins low	Fruit and veg, lean meat, skimmed milk, nuts	Tartrazine
Cheese & tomato pizza	Protein, calcium, some vitamins	One or two vitamins low	Green vegetables, fish	One of the better dishes
Beefburger in bun	Protein, iron, Vitamin B12	High fat, low in several vitamins	Fruit and veg, fish, potato, pulses, milk, wholegrains	OK now and then
Cheeseburger and fries	Protein, calcium, some vitamins	High fat, low in several vitamins	Fruit and vegetables, fish, wholegrains, milk	May have Azo dyes

Food	Good source of	Poor source of	Serve with	Notes
Cod roe in batter	Protein, many vitamins	Low fibre	Potatoes, green vegetables	May have Azo dyes, but good dish to eat
Sausage in batter	Protein, calcium, Vitamins B3, B12	High fat, low fibre many vitamins low	Fruit and veg, fish, wholegrains, milk	May have Azo dyes
Spare ribs in sauce	Protein, calcium, zinc, some vitamins	Low iron, some vitamins low	Fruit and veg, pulses, lean meat, wholegrains	May have Azo dyes and monosodium glutamate
Spring roll	Protein	High fat, low calcium and many vitamins	Fruit and veg, milk, fish, lean meat, pulses, wholegrains	Not brilliant on its own
Chicken Madras	Protein, iron, zinc	High fat, low fibre and some vitamins	Fruit and veg, pulses, wholegrains	Good with dahl and potato
Lamb curry	Protein, iron, zinc, some vitamins	High fat, low fibre and some vitamins	Potatoes, fruit, pulses, green veg, wholegrains	Good with dahl and potato
Cheese & onion pastie	Calcium	High fat, low in iron zinc and some vitamins	Fruit, veg, lean meat, fish, milk, wholegrains, pulses	Not brilliant on its own
Deep-fried apple pie		High fat, poor on many other nutrients	Full range of nutritious foods	Not brilliant on its own
French fries	Vitamin C	High fat, poor on many other nutrients	Full range of nutritious foods	Not brilliant on its own
Milk shake	Protein, calcium	High sugar, low fibre and several nutrients	Fruit and veg, potato, lean meat, pulses, fish, wholegrains	Not brilliant on its own

Source LFC: Southwark Public Protection.

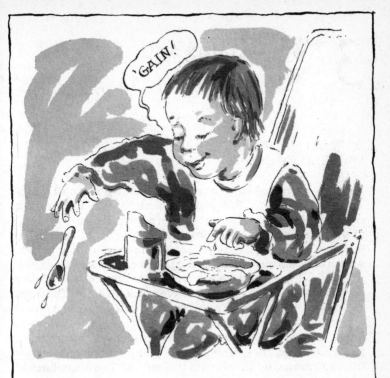

Moll's six months old; she wants her jar
Of runny purée, based on water,
Thickened by starch and one or two beans,
Flavoured by hydrolysed vegetable proteins,
Coloured by beta-carotene and riboflavin
(Aluminium, too, is that misbehavin'?)
O mother, be calm. Though you buy for
                                expedience,
You have bought, to be sure, only
                    natural ingredients!

3 Who Gains and Who Loses?

WHY DO MANUFACTURERS LIKE SELLING PROCESSED FOOD?

Food manufacturers have to consider one thing above all others. They have to ensure that their business survives against other competing businesses. The directors of a company are responsible to the shareholders, and the shareholders purchased their shares with one purpose in mind – to see a good return on their money, with divided payments and a general rise in the value of the shares.

The directors hire managers to run a company, and they choose people best able to see that the company makes a profit. The larger the profit, the happier are the managers, directors and shareholders. This is no great secret: just listen to the business reports on the radio, with the 'good' news about rising share values on the Stock Exchange, the 'welcome' mid-year profit announcements from companies, or the 'nervous trading' and 'loss of confidence' when profitability is in question.

But there is a problem about selling food and increasing profits. you can't simply sell more and more food. We might be sold a second television, or a second car, but we can't be sold more and more meals each day – we have a capacity to the sheer amount of food we will consume before we feel full.

So what can make a food company happy? ADDED VALUE. This means increasing the apparent 'value' of something so that it can be sold for a higher price. Not just bread and meat, but 'Texas-style 100 per cent beefburger in a sesame bun.' Not just apples and pastry, but 'Carefully selected British Bramleys in an individual heat-and-serve tartlette'. It is a matter of taking some ingredients and making them into something that can be sold for more than the cost of the parts and labour. They call it a process of adding value, but really it can take value (such as nutrient value) away and still be marketed for a higher price. Here is an example of the sort of mark-up that manufacturers like to see as they 'add value' to a product (Table 3.1):

Table 3.1 'Added Value' processing can mean added cost
The cost of buying basic foods

'plain' version		'added value' version	
potatoes	15p per lb	crisps	£2.08p per lb
cod fillet	£1.50p per lb	prime fish fingers	£1.60p per lb
stewing steak	£1.35p per lb	take-away beefburgers	£5.60p per lb
cornflour	50p per lb	custard powder	£1.10p per lb
froz. strawberries	79p per lb	strawberry flavour mousse	£1.40p per lb
oranges	36p per lb	whole orange drink	44p per lb

Source LFC.

If they can sell us the foods in the more 'added value' versions rather than in the less 'added value' versions, then we have made their day for them. Whether the food is any better for us is not really relevant to the industrial process of adding value – if it *is* healthier then they can market it on that basis. If it isn't then they will market it on some other feature.

If we look at some examples (Table 3.2) we find that, for the money we spend, we often get less nutrients from the more processed versions of our food.

Table 3.2 'Added Value' processing can mean less nutrients per penny
Nutrients for 50 pence

Food	Amount of relevant nutrient
Boiled potatoes (3 lb)	42mg+ Vitamin C
Potato crisps (3 bags)	15mg Vitamin C
Cod fillet (4 oz)	360ug Vitamin B6, 2.2ug Vitamin B12
Fish fingers (5 oz)	310ug Vitamin B6, 1.4ug Vitamin B12
Stewing steak (6 oz)	35g protein, 6mg niacin
Take-away beefburger (2 oz)	12g protein, 2mg niacin
Oranges (1.5 lb)	230mg Vitamin C
Orange drink (400ml)	1mg Vitamin C (unless as additive)

Source LFC McCance and Widdowson, *The Composition of Foods.*

Table 3.3 'Added Value' processing can mean loading on the calories

Calories per 100 gram serving	
Boiled potatoes	80
Potato crisps	533
Cod fillet	80
Fish fingers	178
Stewing steak	176
Beefburger	264

Source   McCance and Widdowson, *The Composition of Foods*.

But perhaps money is not a problem. Maybe you can afford to get your vitamins from the more expensive sources. But if you rely on the processed versions can you get what you need without harming your health? Or are processed foods inherently unhealthy?

FOOD PROCESSING AND NUTRITION

We can ask whether processing food really makes it any less healthy. Are the useful nutrients that we expect to get from this food still there in sufficient quantity after the food has been processed? Is the food sufficiently rich in useful nutrients after processing compared with before?

The answers are fairly consistent: the calories in an equal weight of the food tend to go up as the food gets processed, and the essential nutrients like vitamins and minerals tend to be diluted with these added calories. To get the same level of nutrients we might have to eat quite a lot more calories (Table 3.3.).

For many people, eating more calories just to get the same level of nutrients is not a good idea. By their mid-twenties, nearly a quarter of the adult population in Britain is judged to be medically overweight, with a greater risk of suffering various disorders like high blood pressure and diabetes. An overweight adult is more likely to have been overweight as a child, so that keeping away from the excess calories during childhood is important.

Besides this, children are in need of vitamins and minerals to an equal or even greater degree than adults: they may need less calories, but they may need proportionally more Vitamin C for example, and iron and calcium. They are not going to do so well if they trade foods which are rich sources of nutrients for foods which are poor sources of nutrients.

A PROFESSIONAL LOOK AT THE NUTRIENTS

Dietitians measure the richness of the nutrients in a food by asking *how much of a nutrient is in the food for the number of calories in that food.* The measure is called *nutrient density.* This is because the human body doesn't need to eat a certain weight of food each day, it needs to eat a certain number of calories. More or less than the optimum number of calories and our body will become over- or underweight. In the food providing these calories our body will need to get all the nutrients it also needs – the proteins, fats and vitamins and minerals – which it cannot make for itself. We also need to get a certain amount of dietary fibre in our food, as this is known to help prevent disorders like constipation and various diseases of the intestine, including, it is believed, bowel cancer, one of the most common forms of cancer in the British population.

Table 3.4 shows the levels of nutrient density needed by young children. It is an *average* for children, remembering that each child will have his or her own metabolism, own appetite and food preferences and own body size, and so will not fit the average exactly. It is useful, though, for comparing foods and asking what foods are as good as or better than these averages at supplying what children need. The figures are based on recommended levels from the Department of Health and Social Security. These figures are for the average nutrients needed spread over the whole day's or even week's food. A 'balanced diet' would mean getting some of the nutrients from some foods and some from others. A variety of foods should aim to reach the average in the tables above.

Relying on processed foods, it can become more difficult to be sure that one's diet is healthy. And it can be very difficult to ensure that one's child, who may be attracted to processed foods, gets an adequate, balanced diet. In Table 3.5 are some foods of the

Table 3.5 Some poorer nutrients-per-calorie foods

Nutrients in common foods, showing whether nutrient densities meet the average needs of children (average nutrient needs per 100 calories, children aged under 5 years).

Food	Protein	Calcium	Iron	Vits B1	B2	B3	B6	B12	C	A
Sugar Puffs	no	no	yes	no	no	yes	no	no	no	no
Spaghetti hoops	yes	yes	no	no	no	yes	no	no	no	no
Frankfurter	yes	no	yes	no	no	no	no	yes	no	no
Sausage roll	no	no	no	no	no	yes	no	no	no	yes
Fruit salad (tinned)	no	no	yes	no	no	no	no	no	no	yes
Lemon curd	no	no	no	no	no	no	no	no	no	yes
Honey	no	no	no	no	no	no	no	no	no	no
Lucozade	no	no	no	no	no	no	no	no	yes	no
Mars bar	no	no	no	no	no	no	no	no	no	no
Dolly Mixture	no	no	yes	no	no	no	no	no	no	no

Source McCance and Widdowson, *The Composition of Foods*.

Table 3.4 Under 5s: average nutrients needed per 100 calories of food

Protein	Calcium	Iron	Vits B1	B2	B3	B6	B12	C	A
2.5g	45mg+	0.5mg+	40ug	52ug	590ug+	70ug	.15ug	1.5mg+	20ug+

+ more than this level is recommended for younger children
Source DHSS.

sort marketed for young children, indicating whether their nutrient density comes up to the level shown in the previous table as the average needed for a child's overall diet. Perhaps no one expects these foods to be really healthy foods, but manufacturers do occasionally promote foods such as these as being part of a balanced diet: we have seen leaflets from manufacturers which show how eating confectionary can help you lose weight if taken as 'part of a calorie controlled diet' (the Mars diet). Yet the foods themselves may do little to help, and might make it even more difficult to get a balanced diet from other foods. Eating these foods gives calories but few nutrients, so that to get a balanced diet means searching for foods which have nutrients but few calories, to compensate.

To show that all is not lost, here are some inexpensive, more nutritious foods (Table 3.6), with nutrient densities that compare well with the average daily needs of a child.

In earlier sections we have seen how our eating habits have changed over the last few decades, and how this has affected the nutrients that we get from our food. But it does not tell us whether this has been a good or bad thing. We have to ask: So what? It's all good for industry, isn't it? What's the problem?

Well …

We need to ask: Who is gaining from these changes, and who is losing? What is it doing for our children? Is there really a health problem?

WHAT'S THE WORRY? WHO IS MALNOURISHED NOWADAYS?

The idea of malnutrition conjures up images of children in poverty-stricken countries showing terrible symptoms of the diseases of starvation. The disease are those of deficiency – a lack of nutrients in the diet. But in the last few decades we in Britain have started to see the results of getting too *many* foods of a certain sort in our diets. These are the so-called 'diseases of affluence', because they are more common in countries that are considered affluent compared with those where starvation is more common.

These diseases are actually more common among *poorer* people in the wealthier counties. The diseases include heart disease and

Some other foods, showing whether nutrient densities meet the needs of average children (average nutrient needs per 100 Calories, children aged under 5 years).

Food	Protein	Calcium	Iron	Vits B1	B2	B3	B6	B12	C	A
Baked beans	yes	yes	yes	yes	yes	yes	yes	no	no	?
Frozen peas	yes	yes	yes	yes	yes	yes	yes	no	yes	yes
Pizza	yes	yes	yes	yes	yes	yes	no	yes	yes	yes
Wholemeal bread	yes	no	yes	yes	no	yes	yes	no	no	no
Puffed wheat	yes	no	yes	no	no	yes	no	no	no	no
Chicken liver	yes	no	yes	yes	yes	yes	yes	yes	yes	yes
Dahl/ lentils	yes	no	yes	yes	yes	yes	yes	no	yes	no
Tuna in oil	yes	no	no	no	no	yes	yes	yes	no	no
Sardines in tomato	yes	yes	yes	no	yes	yes	yes	yes	no	no
Brussel sprouts	yes	yes	yes	yes	yes	yes	yes	no	yes	yes
Sweetcorn canned	yes	no	yes	yes	yes	yes	yes	no	yes	yes
Semi-skimmed milk	yes	yes	no	yes	yes	yes	yes	yes	yes	yes
Banana	no	no	yes	yes	yes	yes	yes	no	yes	yes

Source McCance and Widdowson, *The Composition of Foods*.

diet-related cancers, and diseases related to being overweight such as late-onset diabetes and high blood pressure. There are strong links between these diseases and the eating of foods containing a lot of saturated fats and sugars, and little dietary fibre – such as meat products, fatty dairy food, food rich in hard vegetable fats such as cakes, biscuits, pastry and pies, soft drinks and confectionary – unfortunately, just the cheap and highly processed foods of the sort eaten in large quantities in Britain.

These sorts of food do not cause immediate illness. They are not acute poisons. But they have gradual affects, accumulating over a period of time, until finally something begins to hurt or begins to go wrong and cannot function properly. One part of the body in particular can show the accumulating effects of a bad diet very clearly – our teeth.

When merchants in Britain first started to import sugar from the new colonial plantations, the sugar was expensive and only the rich could afford it. Their teeth began to rot. The result was the development of an unusual industry: denture manufacturing for rich clients. No materials were available for making artificial teeth, so people were offered money to sell their teeth to the denture-makers, and many people who could barely afford to eat at all took the money and parted with their teeth.

As a result of slave labour and the more recent development of sugar beet technology, sugar is now one of the cheapest food commodities available and over 90 per cent of children have tooth decay by the time they are in their teens.

Tooth decay is not the only disease to show itself so clearly. Since the Second World War Britain has seen a virtual doubling of the numbers of men dying of heart disease in their thirties and forties. Heart disease has become the country's number one killer, affecting nearly a million people, women as well as men, and causing a quarter of all deaths. The diet we eat, along with smoking and exercise, is believed to be a key factor in the chance of developing heart disease.

Cancer is another major killer nowadays. According to one eminent specialist, Sir Richard Doll, if we modified our diets we could avoid 40–50 per cent of cancers, especially those of the bowel, breast, uterus and gall bladder.

Being overweight increases the risk of several serious diseases, including late-onset diabetes, hypertension (high blood pressure) and stroke, infertility, pre-eclampsia and death in childbirth.

Insurance companies charge higher premiums for overweight people as they are known to be a higher risk group, with a shorter expectation of life.

We can put some figures to how much our poor diets are costing us. An estimated £700m–£1000m is spent by the NHS medical services coping with the effects of our diet. A further £500m is spent on dental services. Over 35 million days each year are taken off work for diet-related sickness, not counting the days taken and not certified, and the part-days taken for dental treatment.

As well as this enormous cost to society, we spend an estimated £88m on dietary supplements such as vitamins and minerals, and further untold millions of pounds buying treatments for constipations and piles. Many of these costs could be reduced or avoided altogether.

WHEN DOES THE ROT SET IN?

What does this catalogue of today's dietary problems mean for young children? It means quite a lot. First, the habits and attitudes that lead to a bad diet start young. Secondly, the dietary diseases themselves start young.

American teenage soldiers killed in combat were found to have the early stages of heart disease already apparent in their arteries and veins. The blood pressure in children under 10 years old is highest compared with children growing up in traditional non-Western societies. And there is even some indication that early signs of cardiovascular trouble can be found at a very early age, with plaques and fatty streaks in the arteries of children as young as a year or two old who are being brought up on our 'modern' diets.

Teeth show damage from quite an early age, too. Over half of Britain's young children have tooth decay before they lose their first set of teeth. Ninety per cent of children will suffer tooth decay in their second set of teeth while still in their teens.

Untold numbers of children suffer from constipation and the early stages of haemorrhoids. And millions of children each year are more prone to suffer respiratory infections and other ailments because of their poor nutritional status: studies of children in families with low incomes have found that their diets lack essential vitamins and minerals, they are not growing as well as other children, and they tend to get infections more frequently.

Children may also develop food allergies and reactions to food additives. Allergic reactions to cow's milk and wheat gluten are well recognised in young children, and increasing recognition is now being given to the role of additives such as food colourings and antioxidants in causing problems such as asthma, eczema, skin rashes, sleeplessness, hyperactivity and learning problems. Some children with these symptoms have shown an improvement with an additive-free diet, the change being most marked in pre-school children.

Does Poor Diet Affect Learning?

Two studies of the effects of diet on normal school-children have led to great interest among parents and researchers alike. One, conducted in Britain, was reported in the medical journal *The Lancet* after receiving publicity on BBC television. It found that a group of children aged 12 and 13 showed a significant improvement in one particular measure of IQ if they took vitamin and mineral pills compared with a similar group of children who did not take such pills.

The company that provided the pills for the study, Larkhall Laboratories, took out advertisements in the daily press, including full-page advertisements in the Sunday colour supplements, featuring *'The World's First Teacher Tested Vitamins As Used In Famous School Trial'*. Within days supermarkets and pharmacies found their shelves had been cleared of vitamin supplements by anxious parents.

But according to the people who did the study, the BBC programme was supposed to mention that taking pills was not the best answer to parents worried about their children's diets – it is both expensive and unnecessary. Instead, they felt, it was much more important that children ate healthily.

The second study looked at removing additives and improving diets for New York school-children, stretching over four years and involving over 800 schools. The changes involved eliminating foods high in sugar and eliminating foods with synthetic colourings, flavourings or specific preservatives (the antioxidants BHA and BHT). Before the changes in school meals, the New York schools ranked around an average 40 per cent in national intelligence tests for the whole country. After four years of gradually changing diets the schools had jumped to 55 per cent. Before the changes, the schools where school food was eaten a lot tended to have the worst scores but afterwards the pattern reversed, and the schools where school food was eaten most were giving the best scores.

The researchers conclude that two factors may be important: the effect of the additives themselves and the fact that the additives were in the more processed foods. They felt that the second was probably the most important – that the additives were found in the worst sort of food, and that improving the quality of the food was more important than removing the additives.

Studies such as these need to be repeated in different circumstances and with different measures of the effect of the dietary changes. They do, though, provide pointers towards some aspects of children's diets that may be in need of closer scrutiny.

In summary, dietary illnesses start young. If we take 100 newborn healthy infants then all things being equal, on present figures:

48 would have tooth decay by age 5
90 would have tooth decay by age 15
60 would suffer heart disease in some form
53 would die of heart disease, 8 before they retire
10 would die of diet-related cancer
50 will become medically overweight by middle age
23 will become medically overweight before they are 30
around 1 in 1000 are likely to show intolerance reactions to food additives.

These are the figures if all things were equal, but all things are not equal. Some children are at far greater risk than others. A low family income – and hence a diet based on cheaper foods – greatly increases the risk of developing most of these diseases. Even before birth, poverty and poor diet will predict the chances of the baby being underweight: one study found that the cost of an adequate diet for an expectant mother was likely to be beyond the means of families depending on welfare benefits or on low wages.

A detailed study of low-income families in South Wales looked at whether young children under the age of 3 were getting adequate nourishment. The researchers measured all the food that each child ate over a four-day period, and analysed the food for some of the essential vitamins and minerals the child would need from the food. Compared with the amounts that the DHSS recommends that the young should be getting, many of these particular children were falling way below the average. The researchers suggested that in any group some people will stay healthy even if they eat less than the recommended amounts, but that below 70 per cent of the recommended amount should be thought of as 'seriously deficient'. They found:

- one in six children eating food seriously deficient in *Calcium*
- a third of the children eating food seriously deficient in *Iron*
- half the children eating food seriously deficient in *Zinc*
- over 90 per cent of children eating food seriously deficient in *Magnesium*
- one in six eating food seriously deficient in *Vitamin A*
- nearly half eating food seriously deficient in *Vitamin C*
- nearly a third eating food seriously deficient in *Vitamin B6*
- one in seven eating food seriously deficient in *Vitamin B12*
- one in five eating food seriously deficient in *Folate*

This catalogue of dietary disease and poor nourishment in Britain, especially among Britain's children, could be prevented. As a nation we have one of the worst rates of diet-related ill health in Europe. This need not be the case.

SHOULDN'T SOMETHING BE DONE?

The figures for dietary diseases have been sounding alarm bells among health workers and nutritionists for several years. By the end of the 1970s the government had indicated a modest health education campaign, including a pamphlet with such recommendations as:

> It would be wise to reduce the amount of fat, especially saturated fat, in the diet
> The use of sugar and confectionery should be limited
> Obesity can mean ill-health or premature death . . . a practical way (to prevent obesity) is not to become overweight
> To eat less salt might be beneficial
> *Eating for Health* DHSS, 1978

These rather mild suggestions were coupled with a message to 'look after yourself'. We as individuals were told to take responsibility for healthy eating.

The very same day that the DHSS published their pamphlet urging us to cut back on the fat and sugar in our diets, the EEC announced new incentives to encourage higher consumption of sugar, as a way of cutting the sugar mountains. Shortly afterwards our own Ministry of Agriculture announced new proposals to subsidise butter for the elderly and those on low incomes, to reduce the butter mountain. It appeared to the bewildered consumer that the interests of agricultural production seemed to be taking priority over sensible health policies.

In the early 1980s, the advice became more specific. A committee set up by the then cabinet minister Sir Keith Joseph (the National Advisory Committee on Nutrition Education) concluded that, as a nation:

Sugar consumption should be cut by a half

Fat consumption should be cut to about 30 per cent of daily energy needs, and

Saturated fat should be less than one-third of total fat

Salt should be cut by at least a quarter

Dietary fibre, the roughage found in food from plants, should be eaten in greater quantities: half again the amount we eat at present.

The food industry was reported to be rather alarmed at the implication of these recommendations, as it would mean a major shift from refined, processed foods rich in fats, sugars and refined starches, and a move towards less processed, fresh foods with less meat and more vegetables. Who would buy their processed foods? They wanted the report and the recommendations for improving our diet not to become government policy, and it is interesting to note that the government refused to publish the report with these dietary recommendations in it. The report, commonly known as the *NACNE Report*, was eventually published by the Health Education Council in September 1983.

During this period several studies were published showing particular diet-related problems among low-income families. Low birth weights, poor growth, worse dental decay, and greater chance of illness were all associated with low income. People's diets were lacking in adequate Vitamin D, calcium, iron and folic acid. A government study of older school-children who ate in cafés and take-aways at school dinner-time found that their diets were seriously short of several vitamins as well as calcium and iron. This report, too, did not appear for several years, until questions in Parliament and newspapers forced the DHSS to make a draft available. As the report concludes:

> Older children, especially girls, who ate out of school at cafés, take-aways and fast food outlets, etc., had low intakes of many nutrients from these meals, which were not made up by the foods consumed at other times of the day. Iron intakes were particularly affected but generally the nutritional quality of the diet consumed by these children was poorer than those who took school meals, and among the lowest of all the groups surveyed.
> (DHSS report: R. Wenlock *et al.*, *The Diets of British School-children*)

· The pattern that emerges from all this is fairly clear. We are eating, and our children are eating, too many foods low in useful nutrients. The nutrients we get are embedded in a lot of calories. What we need are foods of higher 'nutrient density' – lots of nutrients among fewer calories. This is particularly important for children, because their growing bodies need a lot of these nutrients, sometimes as much as an adult does, while at the same time they don't need as many calories. So children above all should be getting foods of high nutrient density – lots of nutrients per calorie.

They are not getting this. Who is responsible? The manufacturers say that they only sell us what we ask for – we are free to choose to eat healthily if we want to, they say.

Or are we? Are we able to buy what we need? Do we have the choice that they say we have?

FREE CHOICE?

When we go shopping we are encouraged to feel that we have something of a choice. We can spend a lot or just a little on our food, we can go to one shop or another, we can buy one brand or another, we can look at what we buy and judge whether it is what we want ... and so on. Or is this a fantasy? Are we really able to get exactly what we want?

Let us look at 'free choice' from the customer's point of view, and how we are restricted in our choice by factors we cannot easily control. 'Free choice' makes certain assumptions.

First, it assumes that what we want is easily available:

— that what we need is within easy distance, so that *time* and *effort* to get to a shop is no problem
— that what we want is easily afforded, and we do not have to go without something else in order to eat properly
— that what we want comes in the *quantity* that we need, not too much at once for example, and that it is of a *quality* that we can trust and not adulterated with any unwanted material

Second, it assumes that we can select what we want:

— that we *understand nutritional needs* and know, for example, what nutrients growing children should have
— that we *know what makes a balanced diet* and which foods will provide the nutrients that are needed
— that the *information given* on each food item is adequate and useful and quickly understood.

Third, it assumes that there are no problems preparing the food and eating it the way that we want:

— that we have the *time* to prepare it
— that we have the *equipment and facilities*
— alternatively, that we can *eat out* or buy nutritious take-away food if we wish

THE SAME DIFFERENCE

Sometimes what looks like a wide choice of products is in fact very little choice indeed. Until recently you could not buy a tin of baked beans without at least 5 per cent sugar added to the sauce. Even now you will find it hard to get a tin of baked beans with no sweetener added – if it isn't sugar it might well be concentrated fruit juice – which is virtually sugar in another form – or an artificial sweetener like saccharin, which is not permitted in baby foods.

Unsweetened baked beans are very hard to find. And exactly

the same goes for tinned spaghetti in all its various forms. In hoops, rings, letters, characters or monster-shapes, tinned spaghetti is sweetened. If you challenge the baked bean manufacturers you may get told that the sweetness is essential because the original recipe is the 'Boston Baked Bean' dish, which had sugar in it. You may say 'so what?', but even if you accept such nonsense, the same manufacturers can hadly claim that the tinned spaghetti hoop – a modern invention – has 'always been made with sugar'. The truth is that the sweetness makes the bland product more interesting, and attractive to sweet-toothed children, and that taking the sweetness out may lose the manufacturer their sales. So they don't. And so we don't have the choice of these products being unsweetened.

If you think these are rare examples, then here are some more. Remember the unsalted crisp? For many years they became a distant memory for older people, as the little blue twist bag vanished from the packet, to be replaced with crisps that were already salted. Only recently has the salt bag – a sachet now – been reintroduced, and only then at some of the larger shops.

What about ice cream? Nowadays you can hunt around for healthier versions, and for a price get ice creams with no added colouring. But if you want to serve them up in a cone or a wafer you may be disappointed – there is hardly a shop in the nation that can sell you a packet of cones or wafers that are free of added colouring or free of artificial sweetener (it's usually saccharin).

At last, after years of consumer demand, some supermarkets are trying out tinned sweetcorn without any added sugar or salt. But you can't buy tinned fish like sardines or pilchards without added salt. Or, perhaps more seriously, the quantity of fruit or vegetables *guaranteed free of pesticide residues* is alarmingly small, and the quantity of meat guaranteed free of added hormones or antibiotics is smaller still.

At a different level, we have the new phenomenon of processed foods which look very different but which are made of very similar main ingredients, with a subtly different blend of additives to create the greatly different effect (Fig. 3.1). These two packets have the first same three main ingredients from a nutritional point of view – fat, sugar and refined starch.

The main differences are the added texturisers, flavourings, colourings and so forth. One creates a sweet and frothy whip, the other a savoury and runny 'soup'. But the nutrition is similar, and

INGREDIENTS: MODIFIED STARCH, DRIED GLUCOSE SYRUP,
VEGETABLE FAT, DEXTROSE, FLAVOUR ENHANCERS:
MONOSODIUM GLUTAMATE SODIUM – 5 – RIBONUCLEOTIDES,
SALT, DRIED CHICKEN, FLAVOURING, ONION POWDER,
CASEINATE, ACIDITY REGULATOR: E340: SPICES,
EMULSIFIERS: E471, E472 (b): COLOURS: E150, E104,
ANTIOXIDANTS: E320, E310.

INGREDIENTS: SUGAR, MODIFIED STARCH, PALM KERNEL & SOYA BEAN OILS
(HYDROGENATED), EMULSIFIERS (E477, LECITHIN), GELLING AGENTS (E339,
E450a), CASEINATE, LACTOSE WHEY POWDER, FLAVOURINGS, COLOURS (E122)
BETA-CAROTENE), ANTIOXIDANT (E320).

Figure 3.1

the chance of creating a balanced meal by having a soup and a
sweet from these packets is near zero. What looks like a variety of
foods is actually a variety of added chemicals with little nutrient
value. The basic foods are essentially the same. So much for
choice.

ACCESS TO FOOD

One way in which food may not be freely accessible is if it costs
too much. The pricing of foods increasingly favours those who
can afford a cash outlay, private transport and a freezer. There are
many popular food items which cost substantially more if you
have to shop locally and cannot get to a large supermarket and
carry it all home. In Table 3.7 are some examples of the different
costs:

Table 3.7 Costs of local shopping

	Large supermarket own brand	Large supermarket leading brand	Corner shop leading brand
Bread (large wholemeal)	47p	51p	61p
Margarine (500 gram sunflower)	45p	63p	75p
Cheddar cheese (1 lb)	1.27p	1.33p	1.81p
Milk (1 pint fresh semi-skimmed)	24p	24p	25p
Frozen fish (7 oz cod fillets)	69p	1.05p	1.16p
Frozen peas (1 lb)	54p	72p	85p
Frozen oven chips (2 lb)	49p	69p	99p
Baked beans (15 oz tin)	22p	25p	32p
Canned tomatoes (14 oz tin)	19p	21p	23p
Flour (1.5 kg wholemeal)	53p	53p	65p
Macaroni (500 gram plain)	44p	(44p)	60p
Spaghetti (500 gram plain)	39p	44p	45p
Cornflakes (500 gram)	72p	79p	99p
Raisins (500 gram)	44p	(44p)	90p
Sunflower oil (1 litre)	62p	89p	99p
Tinned tuna (198 g)	(59p)	59p	75p
Tinned pilchards (215 g)	(26p)	26p	35p
Corned beef (12 oz)	54p	69p	1.32p
TOTALS	£9.09p	£10.70p	£14.97p

(..) alternative not available
Source LFC.

For many single people, one-parent families, people in short-term housing and very many others, the idea of bulk buying by driving to a hypermarket once a fortnight is out of the question. At least a quarter of all households have no freezer (with over a hundred thousand families having no home to put one in anyway, living in temporary accommodation and classified as homeless). A third of all households have no car. Yet, as the table shows, small neighbourhood shops, that cannot negotiate bulk deals with manufacturers, typically charge 20–40 per cent more than the large supermarket chains. At the same time, their range of products is narrower.

There are well over 4 million families claiming low-income welfare benefits, and a further 4 million estimated to be on similar low levels of income but unable to claim any benefits. Such families are, of course, the very ones who most need to have access to cheap nutritious food and are least likely to be able to get such access. The one reasonable source of nourishment these children could have relied on was the school dinner. But in 1988 the obligation to ensure the dinner had adequate nourishment was abolished. And then the 1988 Family Credit regulations dispensed with the provision of free school meals for many low-income families. What 'free choice' do these children have?

One recent study of people living in homeless accommodation such as bed and breakfast hostels, found that many families could not afford to eat properly. Nearly a third of the women interviewed said that they went without food for up to two days, and one in ten mothers said they could not afford enough food for their children. One woman said she was not permitted to use a kettle and there was no kitchen in the building, so she made her baby's formula with hot water from the tap. Another commented on the problems she had with hygiene: 'How can I keep things clean and sterile when I am washing and preparing food in the same sink I have just washed a baby's nappy in?'

IS POOR DIET JUST IGNORANCE?

Do people know what is good food to buy – what will be good for them to eat and nourishing for their children? Interestingly, the answer is that most people *do* have a fairly strong sense of what is healthy food, and that similar ideas of what is good and bad can be found among families of quite different income levels. There is something of a myth prevailing that the reason for bad diets is that poorly educated people are ignorant of what they should and should not buy. Recent studies of how low-income mothers feed their children have found that although they know what is good for their children to eat, the prevailing circumstances of their lives makes it very difficult for them to fulfil the intentions they set out with. Costs, convenience, and the 'child-appeal' of less healthy foods works against their better judgements.

Further evidence that people are *not* ignorant about what is sensible to eat comes from studies of how low-income families spend their money. Although foods eaten outside the home are not monitored very accurately, the foods that are bought for eating in the home are surveyed continuously by the government. From this survey – the National Food Survey – it is possible to examine the patterns of spending by families on different incomes, and it is now fairly well established that within their limited means *low-income families actually spend their money more sensibly* – in terms of the nourishment they get for their cash. People on a low budget tend to get more 'nutrients per penny' than those on a higher budget. Whether this still gives them *enough* nutrients overall can be questioned, but within their means, people on low incomes are not acting foolishly or out of ignorance.

Knowing what you ought to eat is not the same as being able to recognise it and buy it, though. The traditional way of judging food is through experience of its appearance and taste. In relatively unprocessed foods the appearance and taste can still be a fairly good guide to its quality, though modern storage and preservation techniques tend to make even stale vegetables appear fairly fresh and wholesome. But generally, poor quality unprocessed food can be seen to be poor quality quite easily.

When it comes to processed food, though, there is a major separation between what the food appears and tastes like, on the one hand, and its nutritional quality, on the other. We can't easily see from the picture on the packet of the food inside whether the food is wholesome. And nowadays processed food takes over three-quarters of our shopping budget.

EATEN BY MANY, CONTROLLED BY A FEW

One way manufacturers have of ensuring that you buy more of their products, even if you still don't eat any more food, is to cover the supermarket shelves with different versions of the same thing. We saw in a previous section that we might not have as much choice as we thought we had. There is a reason behind this which needs to be looked at. Might it be that all the products are actually made by the same people, with different labels stuck on to make it look different?

In a typical grocery you might find several different brands of margarine. Here are some common examples:

Flora, Krona, Outline, Blue Band, Summer County, Stork, Echo, Elmlea, Tomor, Delight.

How many different companies actually produce these spreads? The answer is surprising: just one, Unilever (which owns Van Den Berghs).

Here are some names of different sorts of packaged bread:

Mother's Pride, Hovis, Windmill, Nimble, Country Pride, Champion, Sunblest, Mighty White, Allinson, Vitbe, Sunmalt and Hibran.

How many companies produce this range of bread? Just two. Allied Bakeries owned by Associated British Foods, and British Bakeries owned by Ranks Hovis McDougal.

Of course, we find in all walks of life that large companies get larger, and buy up small companies, and so perhaps we should expect some brands to be owned by others. But for just one or two companies to dominate the whole of a particular section of the food market is quite unusual. It doesn't just happen by chance.

One of the tricks that a company uses to try to put its rival out of business is deliberately to create new brands of virtually the same product. Each brand will get a space on the shelf, and so will squeeze the others. For example, if you wanted to sell jam, you would be well advised to sell six different brands of jam instead of one: this will take up quite a lot of space on the grocer's shelf, and leave little room for your competitor's product. That's the way to dominate the jam section. The fact that the consumer gains very little by being offered six different makes of the same thing is not what worries you, as long as the stuff gets sold.

Having come to dominate one part of the grocery, you turn your attention to others. Several different sorts of food may actually be owned by the same parent company. For example, here is a list of makes:

> Batchelors, Vesta, Surprise, Farrows, Bird's Eye, Brook Bond, PG Tips, Red Mountain, Fray Bentos, Oxo, Haywards, Beanfeast, Lipton, Marine Harvest, Mattesons, Wall's, Richmond, John West

All these are owned by just one company: Unilever, who also own the margarine brands we mentioned above, and several dozens of other products and companies, too. The company is one of the largest in the world. As the box shows, the company's annual sales are greater than the entire economy of several countries, even that of Ireland.

Several companies with food interests have sales exceeding the entire economies of whole countries. Here are some examples:

Table 3.8   Comparing food companies and national economies

Annual turnover/Gross Domestic Product		
Unilever	£16,693m	(1986)
Safeway (USA)	£13,729m	(1984)
General Foods (USA)	£6352m	(1984)
Pepsico (USA)	£5240m	(1984)
Imperial Foods	£4381m	(1984)
Marks and Spencer	£2854m	(1984)
McDonald's (USA)	£2826m*	(1986)
J. Sainsbury	£2576m	(1984)
Tesco	£2277m	(1984)
Cadbury-Schweppes	£1703m	(1984)
Eire	£12,287m*	(1985)
Ghana	£3240m*	(1985)
Ethiopia	£2820m*	(1985)
Mozambique	£2153m*	(1985)
Bolivia	£1987m*	(1985)
Nicaragua	£1907m*	(1985)
Jamaica	£1320m*	(1985)
Malawi	£647m*	(1985)

*converted from dollars to sterling @ 1.5:1
Sources   Company Annual Reports; *Times 1000*; World Bank.

In summary, many of the products we are offered on the shelves of our shops are produced by just a few, very powerful companies. The decisions that just a few senior executives make affect thousands of us, yet their decisions are not made public. What sort of free choice do we have about their decisions?

THE LAW AND CHOICE

These large companies are under one set of pressures: those of their shareholders who expect a good return on their investments. They are not answerable to any other set of pressures – except the law of the land. But how far does the law protect us when it comes to ensuring that food is of good quality? Can we be sure that when we make our choices, we are choosing between products of good quality, regulated by the law?

Up until 1986, meat products were tightly controlled by food regulations. If a product said it was beef in gravy, then it had to *be* beef in gravy, with a major part of the product beef, and a lesser part gravy. But in 1986 the meat standards regulations were abolished in large part, and for many products it was no longer necessary for manufacturers to include specific minimum quantities of meat. Now, in the name of 'giving the consumer greater choice' the manufacturer can include as much or as little meat as he pleases, and still call it meat in gravy. The only requirement is to say somewhere on the label how much meat is in the product (and a third of *that* can be fat, although it doesn't have to be mentioned on the label).

So now you can find canned meat products with as little as 15 per cent or even just 10 per cent lean meat in them. A survey by Shropshire Trading Standards officers found that of a sample of twenty-two products, every one had less meat in it after the regulations were abolished, and that the average loss was over a third of the meat content.

A hurried shopper may not stop to read the label very carefully, and may not think too hard about the quantity of meat that might be expected in a can. A loss of a third of the meat might not easily be noticed. Is this what is meant by free choice?

THE NEW ADULTERATION

Food quality, food hygiene and anti-adulteration laws have been in existence in Britain since the thirteenth-century Bread Assizes introduced weights and measures acts regulating the weights of goods being sold and making it a criminal offence to sell short measures. There followed various regulations preventing people selling food that was going bad or that was not what it claimed to be. In pre-Victorian England several notorious cases of food adulteration were uncovered, such as water in the milk, bone powder or plaster of paris in the bread, sand in the sugar, brick dust in cocoa, and tea leaves made of birch and ash leaves or even made out of used tea-leaves recoloured with graphite or copper.

Despite the publication of widely read reports on the poor standards of food and their widespread adulteration, the government took little action for some forty years. Not until 1860 was the first Food Act passed, and even then it was several years before the adulterations began to decline. Twelve years later, it became an offence to add ingredients that made the food larger or heavier without declaring that you had done so.

Where are we now? Are our foods so tightly regulated that no similar adulterations could occur? With many thousands of processed foods available now that were unknown just a few decades ago, let alone when the food acts were first drafted, are we better protected than our Victorian ancestors?

TRADE TACTICS – 'IT'S ALL LEGAL, GUV!'

Food producers have various tricks up their sleeves to make food appear to be more than it is: more appetising, better value, leaner, fruitier, more nutritious and generally better quality than it actually is. They have available a range of chemicals and processing techniques which can manipulate the raw ingredients in to ever more wonderful products.

All these are permitted by law. The food regulations only require that a manufacture does not claim that the food is something different from what it is. Here are some examples taken mostly from the meat trade showing the tricks that manufacturers can use, and many do use, and yet still say within the law.

Tactic 1   Add water

- Regulations now allow cooked meat to have as much water in it as the raw meat it came from, without anything being put on the label to say this unexpected water is there. Ready cooked cold chicken on the meat counter at the supermarket can have, say, 15–20 per cent water added to it with no need to tell us – far more than it would have if we had cooked it ourselves.
- In the dairy trade, regulations now allow dairies to have up to 3 per cent added water in our milk. For families taking a couple of bottles of milk every day, that could mean nearly a pint of pure water every fortnight.

Tactic 2   Cut the lean meat

- One way of extending meat is to add fat. You can still call it meat on the label, but providing you don't overdo it you can get away with quite high fat levels in meat products. An economy burger can be less than a third lean meat, with the rest fat, water, soya, and what have you. A 4 oz jumbo beef sausage can be 1 oz of lean, 1 oz of fat, and 2 oz of bread and water. Yet the word fat need not appear on the label. And recent relaxation of the regulations now allows various products, like canned meat and various other meat products, to put whatever fat they like in the product without having to say how much fat there is.
- Furthermore, other animals can be used: canned beef mince may have chicken or turkey in it, beefburgers can have a percentage of pork meat, for example, and there need be no indication of what meat has been used.

Tactic 3   Use cheaper ingredients

- Bulk out the expensive items with cheap ones, just as they used to do. It is now quite legal to put bread or flour in meat products and still call them meat: sausages, saveloys, burgers – all are likely to have added rusk, soya flour, modified starch or wheat flour. These serve to soak up the water and fat, keeping the mixture 'firm and meaty'. Perhaps even cheaper, and quite legally found in our food nowadays, are the thickeners and stabilisers obtained from seaweed, wood pulp and by-products of the cotton industry.

- Use the cheaper cuts: recent changes in the law have made it clear what is and is not allowed to be called lean meat. All these are lean meats:

Mammals: diaphragm, head muscles, heart, kidney, liver, pancreas, tail meat, thymus, tongue, skin, rind, gristle, sinew;
Birds: gizzard, heart, liver, neck, skin, gristle, sinew.

There are more items that can also be used, but if they are used then they should be put on the label:

Brains, rectum, feet, spinal cord, intestines, spleen, stomach, testicles, lungs, oesophagus, udder.

This isn't much good to consumers when there is no label to read. Where is the label on restaurant food, or take-away food? Where is the label on pies and pasties bought loose in a bakers? Can you read the labels at cold counters and delicatessen counters?

- When it comes to margarine and butter the composition of these products is tightly controlled by regulations. But the new 'butter and vegetable oil' mixes are not controlled by the regulations, and nor are the 'low-fat spreads'. The first of these can get away with selling cheap vegetable fat at nearly butter prices, and the second can get away with selling even cheaper water at margarine prices.

Tactic 4   Don't let any meat escape

- New methods of getting meat off bones at the abattoir means that we can now enjoy MRM: Mechanically Recovered Meat. Carcasses which have been stripped of meat by the usual means (knives) can now be massaged and spun under pressure to force the remaining bits of meat, gristle, sinew and marrow off the bones, to form a liquid meat slurry. This is called MRM and can be added to meat products as if it were regular meat. The only problem is that it needs thickening, colouring and texturising to make it look and feel like meat rather than grey soup.
- Another way of not letting meat escape is to return the misshapen and unsaleable products back into some other form. Several meat products make use of this economic

method of recycling meat that might otherwise get wasted. This is the industry's definition of pork luncheon meat:

'Luncheon meats usually consist of finely chopped meat and fat, with or without some added cereal and water, cured with salt and nitrite and heat processed. In practice they are often made in the factory as a means by which meat trimmings and sound edible materials which have been rejected for other products (for instance, mis-shapen pies) may be incorporated into a simple, easily made and saleable product.' (*Food Industries Manual*, 1984)

Tactic 5   Disguise the results

● Never before has the food industry been offered so many tempting products by the chemicals industry. For sale in the catalogues are several dozen means of retexturising food into something quite different. What used to be gristle and sinew can now be chopped finely and then re-formed with the aid of emulsifiers, bodying agents, buffers, firming agents, gelling agents, aerators, neutralising agents, softening agents, suspending agents, thickeners, gums, stabilisers and coagulants, to form steaklettes and burgerettes by the ton. No more chewy lumps in the meat. It is all ground fine and reshaped to look quite different.

● That isn't all, of course. The result would look grey and taste dull, so in go the colours of which there are nearly fifty to choose from and mix how you wish. And in go the flavourings of which there are believed to be several thousand, and in go the flavour enhancers like monosodium glutamate. And of course in goes salt and sugar, vinegar and herbs, till you just can't tell any more ...

● Another way of disguising the origins of the food is to use new types of machinery. There are various gadgets available. An extruder is like an old-fashioned mincing machine, forcing a product out through a set of narrow holes, but in the case of the industrial version this is done at very high pressure, and the result is that the product gets hot just at the moment it is being forced through the hole. This form of instant cooking can create a long string-like product which (according to the size of the hole, the consistency of the mixture, the pressure forcing it through, etc.) can be a fine thin thread, a thicker string, or fat ropes and 'boneless rolls' of instant food.

- A second method which advanced food science now brings us is 'comminution' which means the fine chopping and grinding of any bits and pieces which are fed to the comminuting machine, out of which comes a fine paste ready for emulsifying and texturising, or putting through the extruders. What we end up with are fibres, chunks, hunks, pellets, rolls and so forth that can be easily turned into familiar meat products, like imitation escalopes and steak, with the appropriate moulding and chemical texturising.
- A third way of disguising the results is to make it into a soup. Virtually anything could be put in soup, and we would barely know the difference. Very little meat gets in, even into supposedly meat soups. Here is a manufacturer's recipe for instant chicken soup (Table 3.9):

Table 3.9   Instant chicken soup?

32 %	modified starch
14 %	dried glucose syrup
11 %	salt
10 %	dried onion
9 %	hydrolysed vegetable protein
9 %	beef fat
6 %	monosodium glutamate
3 %	chicken fat
1 %	milk protein
1 %	starch
1 %	flavouring
1 %	acidity regulators, emulsifier, dried parsley and preservative

Source   Industry data.

Not much chicken meat here! But it can be sold in a café or canteen as *Soup of the Day – Chicken* quite legally. But what choice did we have on the ingredients of this soup?

WHO CONTROLS ALL THIS?

Regulations which set the standards for the food we eat are made by central government and largely enforced through local authority food inspectors (various departments of a local authority will be involved: trading standards, the old weights and measures department; environmental health inspectors; public analysts). These are the people who have to try to monitor the tricks of the trade and spot the occasions when a food regulation is broken.

Food law enforcement officers work on very low budgets compared with those of the food industry. One estimate suggests that one food item is analysed for every quarter of a million food items that we purchase, amounting to less than 5p's-worth of food analysis for every person in the country.

Put another way, the food industry spends well over £300 million advertising its goods and persuading us to eat them, compared with less than £3 million that is spent having the foods properly analysed. As a result we have very little knowledge of the presence of unwanted chemicals in our food, like pesticides or antibiotics, and very little knowledge of the standards and quality of the food generally offered for sale. Occasionally, samples of foods are analysed by a local authority or a research department – but the public rarely gets to hear of even this small amount of information. Aluminium in baby foods? Don't know. Water in fish fingers? Don't know. Fungicides in fruit, hormones in meat, heavy metals in fish, salmonella bacteria in chickens? We get to hear very little about these important research questions. Only rarely do we get an insight into what is going on.

But without adequate knowledge we start to rely on rumours, and half-understood scientific evidence, and reports which have been rewritten for newspapers. Any theory can gain credibility when the facts are kept hidden, and the lack of resources to get at the truth means that the industry can keep the facts hidden as long as they wish. No wonder we start to believe that our children need vitamin supplements and that colouring agents cause hyperactivity. It is all quite believable, and the food industry has only itself to blame if we go ahead and believe these things wholeheartedly. Our knowledge is hazy. What sort of basis is this for a rational, educated exercise of our free choice?

In these circumstances there seems to be very little choice for us. Either take it on trust that the food we buy is going to be sufficiently nourishing and healthy, or else take a lot of trouble to read the labels carefully and become an expert in food technology and nutritional science.

Obviously most of us, for most of the time, simply take it all on trust. We walk around the shop picking up products that appear to be the sort of thing we think is good for us, pop it into the basket and move on to the next item. When we get home we might have time to look more carefully at the labels and start to wonder at some of the ingredients . . . but then, well, we've bought it now so we shouldn't let it go to waste . . . and into our mouths, and our children's mouths, it goes.

But quite how trusting should we be? As we have seen, manufacturers seem to be able to put claims on their labels which, to put it mildly, seem quite misleading and contradictory. The claims made can be very puzzling, confusing or alarming. They seem to be able to sell us water instead of meat, fat instead of lean, and put pork or chicken in a beefburger. It is all terribly confusing.

If we cannot simply take the manufacturers on trust, how can we spot which products are really misleading us. And what can we do if there are no labels on the food – in bakers and greengrocers, in sweet shops and fishmongers, in cafés, chip-shops and take-aways? And in the long run, how can we see that things are changed for the better? Who should we complain to, who should we lean on, who gives us honest information and how will we find all this out?

It is the purpose of the rest of this book to help readers find their way towards the answers to these questions. In Chapter 4 we shall try to teach ourselves to be more watchful as consumers, looking at the labels on the back as well as the front, reading the writing in small print as well as large. In Chapter 5 we shall look at the possibilities for changing what our children eat collectively, in nurseries and playgroups and in schools. Then in Chapter 6 we shall consider how to make a fuss and how to demand our rights. Finally, in Chapter 7 we shall check our ground rules by looking at the consensus of opinion on healthy eating guidelines for children, look at the everyday sources of good nourishment for children, and check our children's progress against standard charts. The last pages are a proposed 'Children's Charter' which can be the focus for more determined action and the launch of a campaign.

Molly's mum admits she has often colluded
With her two year-old's taste for a bag of
                                                    extruded
Snack pellets. She dreads those visits
                                            to the shops
(Anything to ensure that the whingeing stops).
Processed, puffed up, crisp starch paste —
Fats, sugar, salt and flavour to taste —
Squeezed at high pressure into any shape
                                            you will,
But 'FREE FROM PRESERVATIVES' — Mum takes it
                                            to the till.

4 Getting What You Want

Up to this point, the book has been largely critical of what we are being sold, and what our children are being sold. The intention is to make it clear that some aspects of our present food supply system, such as the labelling laws and the meat regulations, are not working in consumers' best interests. They need to be changed.

Consumers have rights and these rights have to be continually exercised to be sure that they are not lost. As consumers and as citizens, we need to express our wishes, and to make efforts to see that our wishes are heard. We have to formulate what we want, and we have to plan how we are going to get it.

The sort of food our children need should be

> *Nutritious*
> *Delicious*
> *Affordable*
> *Convenient* and
> *Fun*

Getting this sort of food depends on a food industry willing and committed to providing what we want. It may mean putting public health as a priority above commercial profit and share-holders' returns. At the same time, it should not threaten workers' jobs – after all, the provision of food that is actually wanted and needed by people is more likely to lead to job security than working to make a food product that is merely good for today's company shareholders.

Getting the changes may also depend on a government able to express what we want in the appropriate legal framework, and willing to put the resources into ensuring that the intentions are actually put into practice. It may mean a radical upheaval in the way in which governments work with industry, and it may mean changes in the sorts of people it turns to for advice and recommendations on policy. It may mean creating a senior ministry responsible for food production and public health simultaneously – at least the production of food supplies on health criteria rather than on food industry criteria.

At the back of this book we have drawn up a Charter for Children's Food. This can form the beginning of a movement towards better food for our children, and so try to ensure that future generations benefit from the experiences we have had and the lessons we have learnt. But in order to press for these changes to come about we need to educate ourselves. To educate ourselves we need some basic information. The rest of this book is designed to provide this and lead readers towards further material which they may want to investigate.

TEACH YOURSELF TO READ LABELS

Labels can easily mystify us and sometimes they seem to be deliberately misleading. They flash messages across the front which seem to be clear and helpful, but which turn out to be quite different from what is actually inside the packet, or even listed on the contents list. Here are some examples:

'Low sugar'

This is a flash on a packet that has very little meaning on its own. The actual sugar content might be 5 per cent or 25 per cent or even 55 per cent, so the word 'low' only has meaning when compared with some other value – namely a 'high-sugar' equivalent product. An example of this sort of nonsense was given in the case of rusks. The low-sugar varieties were still sweeter than doughnuts, and only served to show how very sweet the regular higher-sugar varieties must be.

One tactic manufacturers rely on is that the list of ingredients is given in weight order, and that by splitting the sugar up into different types they can put each one further down the list, even though they would come further up the list if they were named as one ingredient. Figure 4.1 is an example:

**Semolina, Skimmed Milk with
Vegetable Fat, Dried Full
Cream Milk, Sucrose, Rice
Flour, Tapioka, Dried Glucose
Syrup, Soya Lecithine, Dried
Yeast, Calcium Carbonate,
Vitamins (A, B_1, B_2, B_6, B_{12}, D,
D_3, E, Biotin, Nicotinamide,
Ca-D-Pantothenate, Folic
Acid), Vanilla, Iron.**

Figure 4.1

Bebelac Biski-Crem
Ingredients include *sucrose* in fourth place, and *dried glucose syrup* in seventh place. Combined, the total sugar might well move into third or even second place. The manufacturers do not declare what amount of sugar is added, but they do say on the front of the pack 'Low Sugar'!

But there is one useful piece of information that the manufacturers give us when they say 'low sugar' which we should not overlook. It means there *is* some sugar present, so if you don't want added sugar then you might need to avoid a product with the 'low sugar' claim.

'No added sugar'

This can mean one or two things: either no sweetener has been added, or else some sweetener other than sugar has been added. In many cases there may be no added sweetener of any sort – these are usually the savoury dishes or the pure fruit dishes where one would not expect to find added sugar anyway. The fruit is sweet enough, with its own 'natural' fruit juice providing the sweetness in the form of fructose (fruit sugar). The savoury dishes are not usually ones where we would expect sweetness to be added, but it is interesting to note that until frequently nearly all dishes, savoury and sweet, *did* have added sugar, and it is only the fuss that has been made in the last few years that has forced manufacturers to remove the sugar.

✳✳

LESSON: CONSUMER PRESSURE CAN SUCCEED IN GETTING BETTER FOOD

✳✳

Another tactic, though, is to add no sugar but to add food ingredients which are themselves very sweet. One example of this is where concentrated fruit juice has been added, e.g. to a peanut butter, but the label says 'no added sugar'. A further example is to add *dried fruit or dried fruit pulp* as some weaning foods do, and yet they, too, put the 'no added sugar' flash on the packet. In both cases the added ingredient is quite a concentrated form of fructose, a fruit sugar which has the same calorie count, and the same potential to damage teeth, as ordinary white sugar.

In some 'no added sugar' cases there are other ingredients which are sweet and which are called by a name other than sugar. The label may be technically correct, but the implication – that there is no added sweetness, or no added empty calories – does not follow and in that sense the label can be misleading. Examples of the names for sweeteners which sometimes appear on the label instead of sugar are given below.

Sucrose   This is actually what we usually mean by sugar – the pure white stuff as well as the brown and fancy sorts.

Glucose   This is what your stomach turns sucrose into. It is just as fattening and tooth-rotting, though not so sweet.

Dextrose   Identical to glucose.

Glucose syrup, dried glucose syrup, corn syrup   These are mixtures of glucose and some other sugars in a syrup (or dried syrup powder). They, too, are fattening and likely to be just as tooth-rotting as glucose.

Hydrogenated glucose syrup   This is a product in which some of the glucose has been converted into sorbitol (see below). It will have about as many calories as sucrose, but is apparently less harmful to teeth.

Fructose   Found naturally in most fruits, and manufactured from corn starch, it is sweeter than sucrose and so less of it is needed to have the same sweet effect. For this reason it can be thought preferable, but in the end it is really no more than yet another form of calories with few nutrients, and just as likely to damage teeth.

Lactose   This is a sugar found in milk. It isn't very sweet and there isn't very much in normal cow's milk or human milk, and the milk itself helps reduce the tooth-rotting effects anyway. But lactose as an added ingredient in food is much like the other sugars, and furthermore can cause adverse reactions in people who are lactose intolerant or have a milk allergy.

Honey   This is a mixture of glucose and fructose, with water and a few traces of nutrients. The glucose and fructose are just as fattening and bad for teeth in the form of honey as they are in any other form, though perhaps the flavour of the honey makes them more attractive.

Invert sugar   This, too, is a mixture of glucose and fructose and so will be just as fattening and tooth-rotting.

Maple syrup   This is mainly sucrose and water, so not much better than ordinary sugar.

Golden Syrup   A trade name for a lightweight treacle or inverted sugar syrup, it is a mixture of sucrose and other sugars, and has much lower levels of useful nutrients than the dark treacles. Just as bad for your teeth and fattening as most other sugar forms.

Molasses, Dark treacle   Although mostly made of sucrose, these do have some useful amounts of minerals (iron and calcium) and B vitamins, but other foods can give you these without the sugar.

Sorbitol, mannitol, xylitol　These are sweet-tasting complex sugar alcohols which can be made from plant material such as seaweed, beet and wood pulp (xylitol is reported to be a birchwood by-product of the plywood industry) or manufactured from sucrose or starch. They are less harmful to teeth than other sugars and are absorbed differently so are less hazardous for diabetics. But they are 'empty calories' in the same way that sugar is, and being a bit less sweet they can mean eating even more such calories to reach the same level of sweetness as regular sugar.

In essence, many of these products are just as much a cause for concern as sugar itself. They are likely to have one or more of the properties that nutritionists are unhappy about:

- they provide a lot of calories but few nutrients
- they can act in the mouth as a tooth-decaying agent
- they make the food sweet and so might encourage a liking for sweet foods generally.

Besides these sugars and sugar-relatives there are various other substances which manufacturers are likely to use, which have the properties manufacturers like but which aren't strictly sugars. These include *starch, modified starch, dextrin and maltodextrin* which help a powder to run smoothly, help a food to thicken when made up into a wet mixture, and which generally bulk out the food with extra weight and volume at low cost. These highly refined and processed *starches and dextrins* have similar properties to the sugars listed above: they, too, provide nutrients in the calories, they decompose in the mouth into sweet-tasting sugars, and they may then also act as tooth-decaying agents.

'No artificial sweeteners'

Artificial sweeteners are the synthetic chemicals like saccharine, aspartame (NutraSweet) and acesulfame which taste sweet but which have few or no calories. To say that a baby food has 'no artificial sweeteners' is the sort of claim that every manufacturer of baby foods and baby drinks can make, simply because *artificial sweeteners are banned from foods specially prepared for babies and young children by law.*

In this case, the manufacturers are simply advertising the fact that they are not breaking the law – which is hardly reassuring for those occasions when they don't say anything!

This is a list of the sugar-substitutes banned from baby foods:

Aspartame (marketed as NutraSweet) (dangerous for phenylketonuria sufferers)

Saccharin   (linked to bladder cancer in laboratory animals)

Acesulfame

Hydrogenated glucose syrup

Sorbitol (E420), mannitol (E421), xylitol

Isomalt   (may have unwanted laxative effect)

Thaumatin

'No added colours'

The same thing applies here: as of 1987–8 *added colours are banned from baby foods by law*, with the exception of three colouring agents which are also vitamins.

Colours (which are also vitamins) allowed in baby foods
Riboflavin (E101) – an orange-yellow colour which can be extracted from natural sources or manufactured synthetically. It is a vitamin, Vitamin B2.

Riboflavin-5′-Phosphate (E101a) – a yellow colour obtained from chemically treating Riboflavin (E101). It is another form of Vitamin B2.

Carotene (E160a) which comes in the form of Alpha-Carotene, Beta-Carotene and Gamma-Carotene, yellow, orange and red versions of similar chemicals. These can be obtained from plant sources (e.g. from alfalfa, carrots, green leaves and butter) or in the case of Beta-Carotene it can be manufactured synthetically. They are chemical relatives of Vitamin A.

Manufacturers can still use these three colours, so there is still the possibility of misleading us, making an egg custard, say, appear more 'eggy' than it really is by adding these colourings. Or else they may use other ingredients which give the product a colour that would not otherwise be there – for example, adding carrot or beetroot purée to a meat dish can make it look as if there is more lean red meat than there really is, and blackcurrant is a powerful colouring agent in fruit dishes.

Apart from these, no other colouring agents – artificial or 'natural' – should be used in foods designed for babies and young children. What are we to make, though, of manufacturers who put on their baby food products 'no added colours' – which amounts to telling us in large colourful writing that they are obeying the law?

'No artificial colours'

This might be more alarming, as it could be taken to imply that there *are* colouring agents present, even though they are not artificial. As the law now stands, no colouring agents should be present, artificial or natural, in foods sold as baby or infant foods (apart from the three vitamin colours mentioned in the last paragraph). So this one needs looking at carefully.

Sometimes a colour creeps in under another name. Caramel might be listed in the ingredients, for example, without it being admitted that the presence of caramel is to serve as a colouring: in which case it could be one of several forms of chemical derived from sugar treated with ammonium salts, sulphites, acids or alkalis, and which do not all carry an entirely clean bill of health. Sometimes colouring is added by adding an extra ingredient to the foods, just to ensure that the colour looks acceptable: grape skin extract might be added to a fruit juice to ensure that the colouring is a deep enough red or purple. Without the extra ingredient the 'juice' might look rather pale and weak (perhaps because it *is* weak compared with the original food).

Both the caramel and the grape-skin extracts are considered to be 'natural' colours. So too is E120, cochineal, a red colouring agent found in the eggs and ovaries of the cactus beetle, a Mexican insect. Perfectly natural to eat insect juice, isn't it?

'No flavour enhancer'

Same as before: *flavour enhancers are banned from baby foods by law*. They should not be in any baby foods. Here is the list of flavour enhancers defined in the regulations (note they have a number but not an 'E' in front, as they do not yet have approval from the European Commission):

620   L-Glutamic acid
621   Monosodium glutamate
622   Monopotassium glutamate
627   Sodium guanylate
631   Sodium 5'-Ribonucleotides
636   Maltol
637   Ethyl maltol

On the other hand, there are several food ingredients which aren't *technically* called flavour enhancers, but whose purpose in the food is to enhance the flavour of what is there. Both sugar and salt can serve these purposes, as can acids like citric acid, lemon juice, vinegar or acetic acid. Then there are various extracts and by-products from other industries such as yeast extract, hydrolysed vegetable protein and meat extracts. They can all be used to boost the flavour, to make the whole recipe more 'tasty' or 'meaty'. They can all give the impression that better quality ingredients were used, or that more of the high cost ingredients are present than is actually the case.

'No preservatives'

Some preservatives are *not permitted by law in baby foods*. These are the nitrates and nitrites which be found in cured meats (E249, E250, E251, E252). They should not be present in any food marketed as a food for babies and young children.

In other cases, the label should really read 'preserved without a listed preservative' because there are many ways of making a food last a long time without using chemicals from the 'E' number list of preserving additives defined by the food regulations. Concentrated sugar acts as a preservative. So can Vitamin C (ascorbic acid). So can salt, and so can vinegar. If these ingredients are present and are serving a preserving function, then to say 'no preservative' (which might give the impression that the product is freshly made) is a little misleading – there are preserving agents present in the food, but they are not being called by the name 'preservatives'.

Even if there really are no preserving agents in the food, the food may have been treated so that it lasts a long time. It may have been pasteurised or sterilised (e.g. fruit juices), it may have been vacuum packed or stored or packed in a gas (e.g. some wrapped meat products and some fruits). All these can serve the purpose of preventing the food going 'off' while it sits in a warehouse or on a shop shelf. The food might look fresh, and say it has no preservatives, but still it is actually not fresh. The time spent in storage can lead to a deterioration in nutrient levels, yet the pack might say 'no preservatives' encouraging us to think it might be fresh and at its best nutritionally.

'Gluten free'

This usually means that wheat was not used in this product. Gluten is found in the protein in wheat, and to some extent in oats and rye. Corn and rice are free of gluten, and often enough the 'gluten free' promotions are merely saying that rice or corn (or the ultra-refined version of grain called modified starch) has been used instead. Or sometimes it is simply put on all packs with no wheat in them – such as 'fruit salads' or 'egg and bacon dinner', where you wouldn't expect to find wheat gluten anyway.

'Only natural ingredients'

This is a big come-on, as virtually anything must start out as 'natural' in some sense or other. Usually it is taken by the industry to mean that the ingredients were not synthesised in chemical laboratories. Even on this they can stretch a point, and frequently call various additives such as flavourings 'natural' or 'nature identical' when they *have* been made synthetically but can be found in a similar form in 'nature' if you were to look for them.

But what is natural? Arsenic and strychnine can be found in nature, but nobody intentionally adds them to the recipe for a baby's dinner. The sorts of chemicals being called natural come from plants that are just as unlikely in our diet as the plants that give us strychnine or arsenic, or perhaps even more unlikely, given that the word 'natural' can be applied to ingredients found in insects, crab shells, bird feathers, seaweed, cotton and wood. Salt, sugar and saturated fat are all natural, but are not necessarily what we want to buy in a healthy meal. Air and water are natural, but when they are used to make a small amount of good food weigh more or seem much larger, then this is using 'natural' products to mislead us. Chalk is natural, but the fact that in its pure form, calcium carbonate, it is used in white flour and baby foods as a 'dietary supplement' to 'fortify' the food is not advertised.

Fruit 'flavour'

This means there is *no* fruit actually used in the product. But if the pack says fruit flavour*ed* then there is some fruit essence of some sort. And if the pack says fruit flavour*ing* then it could mean either of these.

Fruit 'drink'

A *drink* means whatever it likes, but if it says, for example, apple drink then a proportion of the product should be actual apple. This could be minced apple, just as it can mean minced whole oranges in the case of orange drink. If it says fruit *squash* then it must be at least 25 per cent fruit juice, before it is diluted for use. If it just says fruit *juice* then it should be just the juice of the fruit – but check the ingredients list. It may be sweetened juice, or juice with added this and that.

The word *cordial* can be used in place of the word squash, and so should have 25 per cent fruit juice in them before dilution, *but non-citrus* cordials, such as blackcurrant cordial, need only have 10 per cent fruit juice before dilution. The word 'cordial' can be put on the label in place of the word *crush* in soft drinks which have juice in them and which are ready to drink without dilution. In such a case there must be 5 per cent fruit juice, except there is a lower level for lime cordials, which need only have 3 per cent juice. This all sounds rather complicated, but the intention is that there should be a minimum standard for the juice content of the drinks we are sold, and there should be controls over the names that a product can call itself.

However, the whole of these complex regulations are likely to be replaced with a single requirement that all fruit drinks say on the label what percentage of juice is actually present. This may sound like a wonderful simplification, and for the manufacturers it will be. But for us consumers it means that there will be no legal

Table 4.1   Some products with additives 'prohibited in foods prepared for babies and young children'* (NB: Ingredients for products may change and the list below should be checked against current product labels.)

Food	Prohibited additive
Heinz Macaroni Cheese	Monosodium glutamate (621)
Heinz No-added-sugar Baked Beans	Saccharin
Golden Wonder Pot Noodles	Saccharin, MSG (621), (635)
KP Crisps, Hula Hoops, Crunchies	Saccharin, MSG (621), (635)
Smith's Square Crisps, Quavers	MSG (621), BHA (E320), BHT (E321)
Golden Wonder Wotsits, Ringos	MSG (621), (627), (635)
Safeway Savoury Puffs	MSG (621), BHA (E320), BHT (E321)
Sainsbury Cheesy Nik Naks	MSG (621)
Pim's Toffee Popcorn	Gallate (E310), BHA (E320)
Safeway Digestives	BHA (E320)
McVitie's Chocolate Cake	Sorbitol
Quaker's Harvest Bars	Sorbitol, BHA (E320)
Burtons' Toffypops	BHA (E320)
Bird's ready-made mouse	Saccharin, BHA (E320)
Shape Yoghurts	Aspartame
Bird's Trifle Mix	Saccharine, BHA (E320)
Rowntree's Jellies	Saccharin
Bird's Dream Topping, Angel Delight	BHA (E320)
Robinson's Barley Water	Saccharin
Robinson's Whole Orange Drink	Saccharin
Kia Ora Whole Orange Drink	Saccharin
Sainsbury Blackcurrant Drink	Saccharin
Safeway Sparkling Drinks	Saccharin
Rowntree's Pastilles, Jelly Tots	BHA (E320)
Rowntree's Fruit Gums	Saccharin, BHA (E320)
Macintosh Tooty Frooties	BHA (E320)
Mars' Peanut Treets	Sorbitol
Wrigley's Hubba Bubba Gum	BHT (E321)
Wrigley's Orbit Gum	BHT (E321), Mannitol, Sorbitol, Aspartame, Hydrog. Syrup
Lyons Maid Mr Men Ice Lollies	Saccharin
Walls Starship 4, Strawberry Split	Saccharin
Pearce Duff Ice Pops	Saccharin

*There is no agreed definition of the age limit for this group of children. The DHSS has suggested 3 years old, but the Ministry of Agriculture, Fisheries and Food have said that they usually take it to mean only 1 year old. Effectively, the additive is prohibited if the product *says* it is for babies or young children.

Source   LFC; company labels.

requirements to put juices in these drinks, and the experience of deregulating meat products suggests that the overall levels of fruit juice used in these products may drop dramatically.

Incidentally, something like *whole orange drink* does not mean the drink is made wholly of oranges, but means that the drink includes the whole of the orange – pith and skin along with flesh. This orange mince is sometimes referred to on the label as 'comminuted orange'.

'Not for babies or young children'

No – the chances are you haven't seen one like this! We have shown in the previous pages several examples of additives *not permitted in foods for babies and young children*. And yet, as Table 4.1 shows, many foods which are eaten by children, even young ones, *do* have the banned additives in them. How can the manufacturers get away with it? By denying that the foods are intended for babies and young children, and saying that they are for general consumption by people of all ages. This does not sound too convincing, and we believe it is high time that a prominent flash should be put on all foods likely to be eaten by children, and which contain the banned additives.

A shopper's ready reference

Lastly, here is a light-hearted guide to some of the labelling tricks you may meet:

TRADE TACTICS – TELL 'EM WHAT THEY WANT TO HEAR

Label says ...	*But it might actually mean ...*
Low sugar	Sugar added
Low salt	Salt added
No artificial sweetener	Sugar added
Sugar free	Artificial sweetener added
Naturally sweet	Very sweet ingredients
Natural sugars	Brown sugar
High fibre	Added bran
Nature-identical flavouring	Chemically synthesised flavour
Natural flavouring	Added flavour, including nature-identical
No artificial flavouring	Added 'natural' flavours

Rich in vitamins	Vitamins added
Vitamin enriched	We had to enrich this
No artificial colours	Added 'natural' colours
No preservatives	Indestructible
No artificial preservatives	Added 'natural' preservative
Orange flavour	No real orange in this
Whole orange	Pith, skin and all
Succulent	Added water and fat
45 per cent meat	30 per cent lean meat
Other meats	(Don't think about this . . .)

'E' FOR HARMFUL?

When the regulations were drawn up for labelling ingredients, manufacturers were given a choice, they could either state what chemical was in the food or they could identify the chemical using a number – the famous *E number* list of chemicals with their appropriate, European-approved code number.

Gradually, shoppers began to realise that these E numbers were not very informative, and began to suspect that they were hiding a list of unsavoury or undesirable ingredients. Consumers began to turn against products with long lists of E numbers, on the assumption that some, if not all, of these might be harmful or hazardous to people eating them. No one was going to carry the whole list of numbers and their proper names around to see which were good and which were bad, so just anything with an E in front, and any other number, too, came under suspicion.

Manufacturers had only themselves to blame. Putting codes instead of facts on a label does not inspire confidence in what the actual facts might be. Instead, it starts rumours and doubts and half-understood ideas about what was good and what was bad. A good example of the sort of rumour that can catch on is the so-called Villejuif (or Chaumont) list. This was a list of E numbers stating which were harmless and which were dangerous, claiming to come from these named and perfectly respectable French medical institutes. The lists were photocopied and circulated by many people, who were keen to seize on some – any – authoritative-sounding information. Although the French institutes and the French government denied that the list was authentic, the very fact that people took it, photocopied it, passed it to their friends, and felt it was important says a great deal about the food industry and our trust, or lack of it, in food manufacturers.

✳✳

LESSON: WE NEED TRUSTWORTHY, INDEPENDENT INFORMATION

✳✳

Here is a London Food Commission list (Table 4.2) which we feel may be useful to consumers if they are concerned about avoiding additives which are known or suspected of carrying risks. The additives we have selected are those recognised by many authors and researchers as being 'not proven safe'. The list is similar to the one in Maurice Hansen's 'E' for Additives: Shoppers Guide with some additional items.

Table 4.2 Additives suspected of health problems

Number	Name or type	Suspected problems
Colours		
E102, E104, E107, E110, E122, E123, E124, E127, E128, E131, E132, 133, E142, E151, 154, 155, E180	Coal tar dyes	May cause asthma, rashes, hyperactivity. Some have been linked to cancer in test animals.
E120	Cochineal (insect extract)	Suspected of causing food intolerance.
E150	Chemically treated burnt sugar	Some forms may damage genes. May reduce white blood cells and destroy Vitamin B6.
E160b	Annatto (tree-seed extract)	May cause asthma, rashes. Poorly tested for safety.
Preservatives		
E210, E211, E212, E213, E214, E215, E216, E217, E218, E219	Benzoates	May cause asthma, rashes, hyperactivity.
E220, E221, E222, E223, E224, E226, E227	Sulphites	May provoke asthma. Destroys Vitamin B1.
E249, E250, E251, E252	Nitrates/Nitrites	Can produce nitrosamines which are linked to cancers. Can reduce blood oxygen levels.

Antioxidants

| E310, E311, E312 | Gallates | May cause intolerance and liver damage, and can irritate intestines. |
| E320, E321 | BHA and BHT | May cause rashes and hyperactivity. Linked to cancer in test animals. |

Emulsifiers, thickeners, etc.

E385	Calcium disodium EDTA	Possible link to liver damage in animals.
E407	Carageenan (seaweed extract)	Linked to ulcers in colon and foetal damage in test animals.
E413	Tragacanth gum	May cause intolerance, and linked to liver damage in test animals.
E416	Karaya gum	May cause intolerance. Is a laxative so might reduce nutrient intake.
E430, 431, 432, 433, 434, 435, 436	Stearates and polysorbates	Possible link to skin and intestines inflammations and possible cancer, and diarrhoea.
E450a, E450b, E450c	Di- Tri- and poly-phosphates	Possible link to kidney damage, in test animals, can have laxative effect.

Flavour enhancers

| E620, 621, 622, 623 | Glutamates | May cause dizziness and palpitations. Reproductive damage in test animals. |
| E627, 631, 635 | Other enhancers | May aggravate gout and purine sensitive problems. |

Improvers and bleaches

| E924, 925, 926 | Flour treating agents | May irritate stomach. Bleaches destroy natural Vitamin E. |

Sweeteners

| | Saccharine | Linked to bladder cancer in test animals. |
| | Aspartame | Possible link to brain tumours. Dangerous to people suffering from phenylketonuria. |

Source LFC.

CLEANING UP THE LABELS

Manufacturers are getting wise to our general suspicion of 'E' numbers. So now they are, as they like to say, 'cleaning up the labels' (but not changing the food inside!) by removing the 'E' numbers on the list of ingredients and putting the chemical names of the additives instead. Just as before, for many people this will

mean confusion and the start of many more rumours and misun-
derstandings.

Putting long chemical names is just another way of disguising
what manufacturers are doing. A busy shopper would need a
degree in biochemistry just to start to fathom the mysteries of
some of these chemical names. Are shoppers supposed to know
that sodium carboxymethyl cellulose (E466) is a by-product of
the cotton industry and helps manufacturers whip up ice cream,
cheesecake, toppings and icings into a lighter, fluffier product?
And are shoppers supposed to know, too, that it can have a
laxative effect, and there is some evidence that cancer can be
produced if it is injected into the skin?

****

LESSON: PUBLIC HEALTH INTERESTS MUST COME BEFORE FOOD COMPANY INTERESTS

****

A book like this one cannot list all the possible chemicals you
might find on a label, and explain what each one is, and what use it
is to us and to the manufacturers. We need, instead, to be able to
trust the food we buy, and to know that the chemicals – whether
in long names or in coded numbers – have been properly tested
and proven to be safe for even the youngest or most sensitive of
children, and that they are in the food for a good reason, not just
to boost sales.

In the long run, we need to press for:

- greater openness from the manufacturers, making them
  explain why they are using the various chemicals, how much
  they are using them, and how they think this will help our
  health;
- action from the government to ensure that food regulations
  properly cover the vast numbers of additives and other food
  ingredients which we may not expect fo find in the packets we
  are sold;
- research on these extra ingredients to discover any problems
  they may cause, including problems they cause when mixed
  with other ingredients or other additives;
- reassurance that no ingredients will be used if there is reason

to doubt their safety. At the moment there are hundreds of permitted ingredients which are allowed in food on the basis that they have not been shown to do harm. We feel that they should not be allowed until they are shown to be entirely safe, and also useful and necessary. If there is any doubt, then the benefit of that doubt should go to the consumer not the manufacturer. Do we 'allow it until it is shown to be hazardous' or 'ban it until it is shown to be safe'?

Until the day comes when these proposals are put into practice, the best we can do is learn what we can about the chemicals which confuse and mislead us. Those that have links with our health and which may lead to ill health are the ones that matter most, and when it comes to babies and small children we may feel we have to be extra vigilant.

The following pages give a guide to the sorts of chemical names which are used on the baby food packets of today. We have picked out those which may have a health implication for a child.

READING THE SMALL PRINT

Besides the large print on the front of a packet which is designed to make you feel the product is just what you want and need, there is usually some small print around the sides or back of the packet which can actually be much more useful in helping you to judge the value of the product inside.

These next pages provide a guide to the small print on the packets, particularly those containing food likely to be eaten by young children.

A glossary of food terms, ingredients and chemical names, likely to be found on packets of baby foods or drinks.

Carbohydrate
This word covers a range of chemicals. The main nutritional component of sugar, starches, and foods such as flour, rice, and starchy vegetables like potatoes and yams, is carbohydrate. The more refined the foods are the nearer they are likely to get to being pure carbohydrate, with few nutrients other than pure calories.

Manufacturers often put carbohydrate levels of the foods on

the packet. This may be helpful to diabetics who need to watch their carbohydrate consumption. But it would be just as useful to them, and perhaps more useful to the rest of us, to have an indication of how much of the carbohydrate is in the form of sugar. Using the word carbohydrate can actually hide the fact that the product is mostly sugar.

One manufacturer tells us that their powdered drink is 92 grams in every 100 grams carbohydrate. You have to look elsewhere to see that the only food ingredient likely to be contributing all that carbohydrate is dextrose, a form of sugar.

Starch, Modified starch, Modified cornflour, etc.

These are starches derived from plants, including potato flour (farina), cornflour (maize starch), rice flour, wheat flour, sago and tapioca. The refined flour can be further processed by chemical means to produce a whole variety of chemical starches with different effects when it comes to thickening and bulking a mixture. Nutritionally they don't have much more to offer than cornflour, usually less, and cornflour is itself a poor source of most essential nutrients.

If modified starch is towards the bottom of a list of ingredients then it is probably only being used to thicken the mix. Its 'empty calories' will not be a major problem nutritionally, though the starch can be converted by saliva in the mouth into sugar, and so add to the hazards of dental decay.

If modified starch or cornflour is near the top of the list of ingredients then it is more likely being used to 'bulk' the food with the cheap starch, giving the food more volume and weight than it otherwise would have. The starch may be replacing more nutritious food, and the extra 'empty' calories will be replacing possible useful calories. In addition, the thickening action of the starch will attract a lot of water, making the food even more bulky and heavy, without adding any extra nutrients. As starches are converted by saliva into sugar, they not only add to the risk of tooth decay but also give the food additional sweetness, although the manufacturers can say thay have put no sugar in the food.

Typical examples of foods high in these starches are instant whips and instant soups. Some jars of baby foods purées are made thicker than they otherwise would be by using added modified starches (see Chapter 2, ready-to-eat baby foods). Some companies are reported to put up to 6 per cent starch into a product, and for years they have maintained that they could not produce the desired consistency without using it. When the US company Beech-Nut proposed that they would reformulate without added thickener, they stated that some of their products would have as much as 25 per cent more vegetables and 50 per cent more meat than before.

As we mentioned with sugar, by using different names for similar substances, they can be put further down the ingredients list. Here is an example of a baby food (Fig. 4.2) where three forms of thickener (in addition to the natural thickening effects of split-peas, tomato purée, beans and potatoes) have been added, so that the amount of water present is not so visible:

INGREDIENTS: WATER, CHICKEN, CARROTS, POTATOES, FLOUR, HAM
SPLIT GREEN PEAS, PEARL BARLEY, TOMATO PUREE, HARICOT BEANS
MODIFIED CORNFLOUR, CORNFLOUR, YEAST EXTRACT
IRON SULPHATE (iron 2mg/100g), HERBS

NUTRITIONAL ANALYSIS OF PRODUCT

	FAT	PROTEIN	CARBOHYDRATE	ENERGY
Per can	1.8g	3.7g	14.5g	360 kj (85 kcal)
Per 100g	1.4g	2.9g	11.3g	280 kj (67 kcal)

Figure 4.2

Dextrin, Maltodextrin
These are similar to the starches. Just like the starches discussed in the last paragraph they, too, are used to bulk out food, and they also help in the smooth running and non-lumpy thickening of mixtures. Like the other starches, they offer little in the way of

useful nutrition, and can be converted by saliva into sugar – giving both a sweeter taste and a risk of tooth decay.

Many packet baby foods have maltodextrin (Fig. 4.3) quite near the top of the list of ingredients. Here are the first few ingredients from two companies' breakfast baby foods:

INGREDIENTS
Flours (oat, wheat,
soya), Maltodextrin,
Sugar, Vegetable fat,
Skimmed milk powder,
Dextrose

Ingredients:

Dried skimmed milk with vegetable fat, traditional swiss muesli
(apple, wheat flakes, oat flakes, hazelnuts, honey, raisins), malto-dextrin, sucrose,

Figure 4.3

These products use dextrins in powder form. If dextrins are moistened and then allowed to dry they form a sticky gum. According to Professor John Yudkin, the gum on the back of stamps is mostly made of dextrin.

Hydrogenated vegetable oil
Hydrogenation is an industrial process in which vegetable oils are hardened so that their melting points and boiling points are raised. This means that an oil is turned into a hard fat for baking, say, or a soft fat like a soft margarine, or fat for fluffing into synthetic creams.

From the manufacturers' point of view, a hydrogenated fat will not go rancid so quickly, and so the product will have a longer shelf-life, perhaps several months. Also a harder form of vegetable fat means it can be used in powders and dry mixes, whereas oils would make these into pastes.

But for consumers, the effect of hardening a fat is to make it more saturated. As we are being encouraged to eat *less* saturated fats in our daily diet it makes little sense to eat fats which have been deliberately turned from less saturated into more saturated.

Manufacturers don't have to say whether the fat they have used has been hydrogenated. If it is a vegetable fat and has been put into a powder then it is quite likely that it has been hydrogenated, or that a very saturated vegetable fat has been used (e.g. palm oil) which is fairly hard at room temperature without needing to be hydrogenated. In either case it may not be exciting news for our health. Many baby food meals in packets have dried vegetable fat, which is likely to be a saturated fat whether or not it has been hydrogenated.

Hydrolysed vegetable protein
This ingredient, also known as HVP, is a bit like yeast extract, but before the salt is added. It is made from vegetable proteins, such as those found in soya beans, which are then treated with chemicals or enzymes to break them down into their basic components – the amino acids.

Manufacturers find these very useful as flavour boosters. They are not listed as a flavour enhancer, or a flavouring, and are not technically an additive in that sense, but their major effect is not as a nutritious food but as a booster to the loss of flavour that the other savoury foods, like meat, can have suffered during processing. So when only a little meat is used, or when the meat has lost its flavour during processing, then HVP may be the answer (in much the same way that a cook may boost a gravy by adding yeast extracts).

In baby foods it can be very useful as a flavour booster, because manufacturers are not permitted to put the usual flavour enhancers, such as monosodium glutamate, into baby foods. But HVP is actually made of similar compounds to monosodium glutamate, and can actually include glutamic acid which is the main ingredient of monosodium glutamate. So if you are keen to avoid monosodium glutamate you may want to avoid HVP as well.

When they are part of the whole original protein, these amino acids are generally fine. But broken into their acids, and separated out so that we are offered unnatural mixtures, may not be such a good idea. Some studies of animals have shown that imbalances of amino acids like these might be linked to brain damage. At Washington University, scientists have recommended that amino acids like these should not be used in any foods likely to be eaten by young children.

Many baby foods have HVP added as a means of boosting the 'savoury' flavour. Examples may be found of the Beef Dinner with Vegetables types of products, where the original meat has had to be dried, powdered and packed to last months or even years.

Reduced iron

This is one of the forms in which iron is added to boost the iron levels of the food. In this form, a powder version of pure iron, like the sort made into fire grates or manhole covers, it is not easily absorbed by our stomachs and intestines. It is far less easily absorbed than the iron in meat and liver, and the iron in breast milk.

Because of fears that the average American diet was short on iron, the US government proposed that more foods should be fortified with extra iron. The plans were shelved, however, following the reports of various blood experts that the levels of iron could get too high, resulting in a rare disorder called haemochromotosis. Excessive intake of another form of iron, iron sulphate, which is added to some baby foods, has been known to kill young children. However, this is at levels over a thousand times higher than that likely to be eaten in the baby foods with added iron sulphate.

Calcium carbonate

Like the reduced iron, this is a form of a very useful mineral, calcium, presented in a way we don't usually expect to eat it. Calcium carbonate is another name for pure chalk.

Chalk is used in many foods as a way of boosting the calcium levels. It was introduced into white flour during the Second World War for fear that the milk supplies would run down, milk being a rich source of calcium. If children are regularly eating cheese, drinking milk or eating yoghurts and other milk products, then they are very unlikely to be going short of calcium. Both breast-milk and infant formula milks have plenty of calcium.

Calcium carbonate, which has an 'E' number – E170 – is useful to manufacturers as it helps mixtures run smoothly and not develop lumps or cakes. It can also be used as a colouring agent, making something appear whiter than it might otherwise be. In the last century chalk and water mixes were added to milk, and sold as pure milk, and because of its potential to adulterate food calcium carbonate is banned in several countries, including Canada and Sweden.

Calcium, often in the form of calcium carbonate and sometimes in the form of *dicalcium phosphate*, is found in many baby foods, even though very few babies would be going short of calcium. High levels of chalk (calcium carbonate) in the diet may lead to constipation. Excessive absorption of calcium gives rise to a disorder called hypercalcaemia, which can lead to calcium being deposited in the kidneys, heart and other organs. This condition is occasionally found in children, and may be related to taking too much Vitamin D. Eventually it can cause brain damage and can kill, but this is unlikely at the levels present in fortified baby foods.

Ascorbic acid
This is the same as Vitamin C. It has an 'E' number – E300 – because it can be used as an antioxidant to stop fats going rancid and stop colours from fading. It therefore suits manufacturers very well. They can add lots of the stuff and claim they are fortifying their product with extra health.

Natural Vitamin C can be found in many fruits and vegetables, and is essential to our health. Embedded in these foods, Vitamin C would be eaten along with many other minerals, vitamins, trace elements and enzymes. Some commentators are reported to be concerned that we might be better nourished by consuming Vitamin C as part of this rich mixture than eating it as a pure crystalline powder, synthesised in laboratories and sprinkled into our food.

Typical examples of foods with added ascorbic acid are the baby fruit juices, baby fruit purées, and baby fruit yoghurts. Manufacturers can claim that they have added the ascorbic acid to ensure that any loss of the natural Vitamin C due to processing and storing the fruit is being compensated for by adding the synthetic form.

But manufacturers are also keen to put it into other baby food products – for example granulated rusks – where it would not be expected if the rusks were fresh. One such manufacturer puts on the packet 'Allows a nutritionally balanced diet' but it may be argued that such unexpected and unnatural forms of fortification can lead to excessive levels rather than balanced levels.

Pantothenic acid

This is the same as *sodium pantothenate* and is one of the B vitamins. It is present in many foods, especially eggs, meat and whole-grain cereals, but not in the highly processed foods such as sugar, fats and oils.

Having too little pantothenic acid in the diet is virtually unknown. There are suggestions that some alcoholics may be deficient, but apart from babies hooked on gripe water, alcoholism is unlikely to be a problem in infancy.

Biotin

Another of the B vitamins, biotin is found in meats, dairy foods and whole-grain cereals. Deficiency is rare though it has been associated with taking antibiotics for long periods.

Many baby food manufacturers add biotin in with the other vitamin supplements, whether it is to be expected in the food or not.

Niocotinic acid

This is Vitamin B3, and can be found naturally occurring in meat, fish and nuts, milk and whole-grain cereals. It may also be called *Niacin* or *Nicotinamide*.

Niacin is one of the vitamins manufacturers are keen to put in the fortified baby foods. Few babies are likely to be short of niacin, especially if they are drinking milk, breast-milk or formula milk. Excessive amounts of Vitamin B3 have been related to depression and to a worsening of diabetes, but these are unlikely in the levels present in baby foods.

Folic acid

This is another of the B vitamins, sometimes called *folacin*, and may be found in different forms (folates). It is plentiful in green leafy vegetables, and in liver and yeast. It is easily destroyed during canning and other forms of food processing.

Baby food manufacturers frequently include folic acid as part of their fortification of baby foods. There seems to be no evidence that excessive consumption is harmful.

Thiamine

This is Vitamin B1, a vitamin found in many vegetables and meats, especially whole-grains, peas, beans, lentils and pork. Refined foods, especially hard-polished white rice and white flour, may have severely depleted levels, and for this reason it is added as a fortifier to all white flour.

A shortage of Vitamin B1 leads to the disease beri-beri, virtually unknown among children in Britain. It may not be needed as a fortifier in baby foods, but none the less it is commonly to be found in the list of added ingredients. There seems little evidence that an excess in the diet is harmful.

Riboflavin

This is Vitamin B2, found in milk and dairy foods, meat, cereals and some vegetables. It is a colouring agent, with an 'E' number – E 101 – and manufacturers are permitted to use it to colour baby foods with this additive. Eating it can lead to the urine becoming a dark yellow colour.

Vitamin B2 deficiency is virtually unknown among children in Britain. Nevertheless manufacturers like to put it in with the other vitamins in fortified baby foods. An excess of Vitamin B2 is unlikely to lead to any problems apart from urine colouration.

Pyridoxine

This is Vitamin B6 and can be found in meats, fish, egg yolk, whole-grain cereals, nuts and some fruit and vegetables. Deficiency is not common, although the importance of Vitamin B6 was highlighted in 1951 when a number of infants developed convulsions. Some medical detective work found that the babies' infant formula contained virtually no Vitamin B6, and as soon as some of the vitamin was given the symptoms disappeared.

Pyridoxine is commonly added to baby foods when other vitamins are added, as part of the fortification that some manufacturers are keen on. Excess amounts are unlikely to cause any problems, although very high levels have been associated with nervous system defects and degeneration of nerve cells.

Beta-carotene
This is a chemical relative of *Vitamin A*, and may be found as an additive in either this type, or as *alpha-carotene* or *gamma-carotene*. Whichever form it is in it can use the same 'E' number, E160 (a). It can be used as a colouring agent in baby foods, making the food appear more yellow, orange or red than it would otherwise be.

Vitamin A itself is often added to baby foods as part of the fortification some manufacturers practise. As Vitamin A is found in full-cream cow's milk, breast-milk and infant formula, and in many green and yellow vegetables, and in liver, it would seem unnecessary as an added fortifier in infant foods. Furthermore, there is some evidence that there are various different forms of Vitamin A which are found in different food sources which do not all have the same effect, it would therefore be unwise to rely on one source – the fortified foods.

The Vitamin A found in green and yellow vegetables is beta-carotene, and is not thought to do any harm even at high levels of consumption. Indeed, some studies have found that the chances of getting cancer are less if foods with plenty of beta-carotene are eaten regularly. But the Vitamin A found in meat and milk does not appear to have this same beneficial function, and might, in large doses, result in pain, sleeplessness and headaches.

Cyanocobalamin
This is Vitamin B12, found primarily in animal-based foods including dairy foods, and in yeast. Strict vegans, who only eat vegetables, may suffer a deficiency of this vitamin. But otherwise there is very little likelihood of a child being deficient, and the value of the vitamin in fortified food is probably minimal. Excessive amounts are unlikely to do any harm, but in its pure form as a fortifier it may worsen some eye problems. Hydroxycobalamin is the preferred fortifier.

Cholecalciferol
This is a form of Vitamin D, usually referred to as D3. Vitamin D deficiency leads to rickets, a disorder fairly rare in Britain, but present in sufficient numbers for there to be care taken among some groups of children to ensure they get enough.

Most children get all the Vitamin D they need from breast-milk or infant formula, as well as from foods such as butter or margarine (which has added Vitamin D), whole cow's milk and fish (oily sorts like herring, mackerel, sardine and tuna) and lastly – but most importantly – from the action of sunlight on their skin. Vitamin D is also present in the recommended vitamin drops available from children's health clinics. The need for it in fortified food is minimal. Too much Vitamin D is related to hypercalcaemia (see Calcium carbonate above).

Alpha-tocopherol

This is a form of Vitamin E, which can be found naturally in vegetable oils, nuts and seeds, and to a lesser extent in dairy fats. Some studies have suggested that it is valuable in helping prevent heart disease, and some less well substantiated studies have suggested it is useful to inhibit muscular dystrophy and slows down ageing.

The quantities a body actually needs are not well established. Deficiencies are not easily spotted, although premature infants may benefit from Vitamin E supplements to prevent red blood cells from breaking apart. There is no evidence that excessive amounts are harmful.

This vitamin is present in plentiful quantities in diets which have vegetable oils, nuts, and seeds, etc. in them. Babies might benefit from supplementation – little is known on this – but not all manufacturers put it into the baby food even when they do fortify the food with other vitamins.

Sodium

Common salt (sodium chloride) is the main source of sodium in our diet. Babies do not need any added salt in their foods, as they get enough from sodium present in food already.

Manufacturers of baby foods used to add salt – mainly to make the food taste more interesting to the adults who were serving it up – but the companies have been frequently advised by government health committees that this is not in a baby's best interests. Now they leave the salt out, and make a virtue of this by flashing 'no added salt' across their packets.

Manufacturers may indicate the sodium level of their product. If they are doing this then they are probably well aware of the need to keep the level low. In which case there is little need to look at whatever figure they give – usually around the 0.1 grams (or 100 mg) per 100 grams level – as it is likely to be well within the bounds of the acceptable.

Phosphorus

Dairy foods, nuts, whole-grains as well as meats, fish and lentils, are all good sources of natural phosphates. It is unlikely that any supplements would need to be given. There are some suggestions that high levels of phosphorus and low levels of calcium in the diets of older children and adults may lead to osteoporosis, the development of weak and brittle bones in older adults.

Zinc

This is a mineral found in fish, meats, nuts, vegetables and whole-grain cereals. There is some evidence that older children can become zinc deficient, but younger children with adequate milk consumption – breast-milk or cow's milk – are unlikely to go short.

Emulsifier E471

This is an additive used to bind fat to water, and so make a whip, or sauce, or give a creamier texture to a product. It may be used to add extra fat and water to a product, making it larger and heavier than it otherwise would be, or it may be used to make a dough more stable with a more even spread of the ingredients throughout the mixture. The chemical can be made from vegetable fats or from glycerin, or from beef tallow. Most packets do not indicate which of these it is from, and so vegetarians and vegans may wish to avoid it, as may those with kosher or halal diets.

Emulsifier E471 can be found in various baby foods, including the teething rusks.

Lecithin E322

As with E471, this is another emulsifier, which can be used to bind together fat and water to bulk out a product, or to hold the fat in a more stable form. It can also act as an antioxidant helping to prevent fat from going rancid and colours from fading, and so prolong the shelf-life of the product.

Most lecithin is derived from soya beans, but some is made from other vegetable oils and some from eggs, milk, liver or fish. If the source is not indicated then vegetarians and vegans might wish to avoid it, as might those with kosher or halal diets.

Skimmed milk powder
Manufacturers love this stuff:

> 'Skimmed milk powder performs three major functions as a
> food ingredient: it imparts a desirable dairy flavour, it
> contributes to food texture and enhances the development of
> desirable colour and flavour compounds. Skimmed milk
> powder is the most widely used form of milk protein in the
> food industry. It functions very effectively in terms of water
> binding, fat emulsification and structure formation.' *Food
> Industries Manual*, 1984

It is also fairly cheap, distributes easily throughout a product,
and looks much better on the label than any of the 'E' numbers
that might provide some of these functions. The fact that
making powdered milk involves evaporating it and spray-drying
it, with a consequent destruction of some of the vitamins, is not
mentioned. Some of the wonderful 'dairy flavour' may simply
refer to the fact that skimmed milk powder is 50 per cent lactose
(a form of sugar).

Malt
Malt is sprouted grains of barley, which are rich in *alpha-amylase*,
an enzyme bakers use for two purposes: first, it gives a 'malted'
flavour which adults find attractive, and secondly, it converts
some of the starch in the flour into maltose (a sugar), which feeds
the yeast and gets the bread rising.
   In baby foods it is present largely for these same reasons – to
help the mixture rise (e.g. a rusk) and to give the final product
adult-appeal. Nutritionally it has very little effect, except that
some of the starch will have become sugar. *Malt extract* is largely
made of this sugar, maltose.

Vanilla
This is a spice, extracted from the vanilla pod. Its presence in baby
foods is to give the food a flavour which appeals to adults. We
have no idea if it appeals to babies, because by the time we can ask
them they have grown used to having it with their sweeter foods,
and may have come to like it for that reason. Like malt, the flavour
is really there to appeal to whoever has the job of feeding the
baby.

Vanillin
This is a synthetic form of vanilla. It is chemically similar, though not so complicated and so not so subtle. It can be made out of waste from the wood pulp industry, and in high doses (3 grams per kilogram bodyweight) it has proved lethal to laboratory animals. (The equivalent dose for a child would be at least three or four teaspoons of the pure flavouring, which is unlikely to be met from foods flavoured with vanillin.)

As with vanilla, when it is found in baby foods it has been put there for one purpose – to appeal to the adults who prepare and serve the food. The food companies know, of course, that adults are the ones who buy the food, not babies!

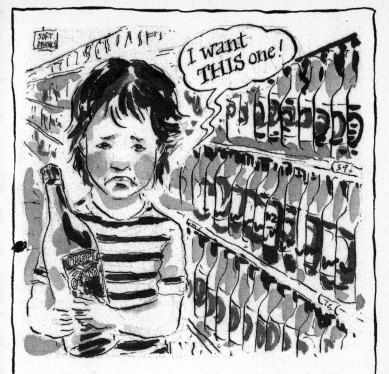

"I want some orange!" cries our Moll at three.
This one looks good: it's 'TARTRAZINE FREE'.
Though water, citric acid and sodium benzoate
With CO_2 and Sunset Yellow merrily congregate,
Mum has her doubts but buys 'whole orange'
                      comminute
Of pith, skin and flesh, thus settling dispute
Between 'orange', 'orange flavoured', 'orange flavour'
                      or 'squash',
Which one has juice in and which one's just trash.

5 It Isn't All Hopeless!

CHILDREN UNITE

The habits and attitudes that lead to a bad diet start young. The diseases themselves start young. As responsible adults we want to see the best for our children and want to know what we should do to ensure that they get the best that we can give. We have looked at how, as shoppers and buyers of food products, we can at least start to read the labels and understand some of the tricks of the trade. We can look out for ingredients which we think are not doing our children any good, and avoid them.

In this chapter we shall turn our attention to the places where children receive food *where there is no label to read* and where parents and guardians are not making the decisions, and yet where young children may be receiving as much as a third of their daily food. These are the playgroups, nurseries and schools, which between them take on responsibility for feeding large numbers of children, day after day. In these organised, collective places of child-care there needs to be even greater responsibility for children's well-being, as so many children can be affected by one person's decisions. The staff in charge make choices which affect all the children present, and even a small change in their approach can have an effect on many children.

Not only do the choices made by staff in these child-caring centres have an effect on large numbers of children, they affect the parents and guardians who use the centres, too. What the staff decide is good for the children, and what the children are encouraged to learn and understand, will affect their home lives. The children will start asking for things they may not have asked for before, and the parents and the adults at home will start to see what is being done for their children during their day-care. More than that, many adults at home will look to the day centre as a place of some authority, and if there are changes being made it must be because changes ought to be made. The children's parents and guardians are seeing what can be done, and seeing the fact that the staff think it should be done.

NURSERIES AND PLAYGROUPS

Over half a million young children are benefiting from going to playgroups in the United Kingdom, and many thousands more attend nurseries which are maintained or registered with the local authority social services departments. That is half a million snacks and several thousand meals provided every day through these day-care centres.

Government guidelines on healthy eating, and the independent guidelines produced by the NACNE committee and the Health Education Council, talked about what constitutes a good diet for the majority of the population. But both reports largely excluded children under 5 from their advice, and gave little alternative to turn to. To fill this gap a report from the London Food Commission, in 1985, outlined some guidelines for staff in charge of under 5s' facilities. Two years later, a report from the British Dietetic Association – the professional organisation for dietitians – studied the needs of younger children and came up with some suggestions and advice. Then in 1988 the DHSS's Panel on Child Nutrition published a new edition of *Present Day Practice in Infant Feeding* with some guidelines on diets for under 5s. These dietary recommendations for young children are very similar, and summaries of them are given later in this book (see Chapter 7).

It is important, though, to realise that we need to go further than simply providing better diets for young children. The guidelines need to be set in their practical context, which for organised day-care means *setting the dietary guidelines in the experiences of nursery and playgroup staff, and the needs of the children.*

This means looking at several themes:

- Food is fun and educational
- Food is part of culture
- Food means work for staff
- Food costs money

These themes are interrelated, so that starting new ideas in one area may well have implications for another area. A play-event focusing on vegetables may lead to more interest in having vegetables for a snack. This has an effect on the budgets, and on the preparation of the snacks. Can we afford it? Is there time for this? Who will do it? It may mean changing the menus, especially when meals need to be worked in around the snacks. It may mean more attention to food hygiene among the children. It may mean that the cook is invited to join in with the play activities.

Remembering that there will be these implications of any changes and new ideas, let us look at the various themes in turn.

Food is fun – and educational too!

One nursery arranged a trip for the children. It wasn't to the local playgrounds or the park, nor even to the local library or the swimming pool. It was to the wholesale fish market. It was a great success. The children were overawed and the wholesalers greatly amused. Several of the children had never before seen fish with heads on. They had only ever seen fish fingers and cod balls, yet there in the boxes and on the marble slabs were fish – and none of them had fingers!

There are many activities which encourage an understanding of the social and environmental context of food. Children could be making models from food packages, for example, or playing guessing games about what might be inside a package judging from the picture on the wrapper. (It is surprising how often the package does *not* give a picture of the actual contents.)

By way of contrast with packaged food, a collection can be made of food that can be found locally growing wild in parks and waste lots, or cultivated in people's gardens. What is food for an animal? What do animals eat that we eat too? Why don't we eat dog biscuits?

Furthermore, as many day centres already know, there are a range of social 'games' that can be played using the play house or play kitchen: a café or snack-bar can be organised which serves snacks at mid-morning break; or a shop selling fruit, for example, or selling other foods – either real or made from playdough, etc.

At one playgroup, twice a week, the children now make their own mid-morning snack. They might prepare chopped vegetables to be eaten as they are or made into a soup, or else made into vegetable juice (the staff use a blender/juice-maker). Or they make dough or pastry for rolls and scones, oat biscuits or muesli bars. They also make bean pictures, using paste to stick all sorts of beans, lentils, grains and pasta shapes onto paper in colourful, textural patterns. There are experiments in growing (and eating) indoor fresh food like bean sprouts, alfalfa and cress. Now they are trying out curry and other spices mixed with paste and painted onto paper as aromatic pictures.

Playleaders and other staff can devise their own visits to markets, allotments, farms and shops to look at the raw materials of our diets, and they can devise their own food-related play materials and snack ideas. Many staff are already doing these things. Here is a summary of ideas for snack foods that are generally nutritious and which can involve children in handling and preparing and having direct contact with the food they may subsequently be eating.

SOME WAYS OF INVOLVING CHILDREN IN SNACKS AND MEALS

Baked apples: cored and stuffed with dried fruit – the children do the stuffing.

Vegetable soup, vegetable juices: vegetables being cut and broken into pieces by the children.

Fruit salads, vegetable salads: again, the fruit or vegetables can be cut and broken by the children. The children might also serve these to each other.

Pasta shapes: these can be used to make pictures, stuck on paper, or to make the contents of rattles, contrasted with rice or bean rattles.

Lentils, dahl, beans: similarly these make good sources of colour and texture on pictures, or stuck on the surfaces of packets, etc.

Spices in the soups, dahls, etc.: these can be mixed with paste to make aromatic paints.

Crackers and cottage cheese: good for making spreads before eating (and fairly easy to clean afterwards).

Bread rolls and scones: these can be home-made by the children – sifting, mixing, adding raisins, etc. (Low sugar and wholemeal flour preferred!)

(continues)

Bean sprouts, cress, alfalfa: Mung beans, alfalfa seeds and cress seeds are fairly reliable as indoor 'plantations'.

Popcorn: uncooked, the corn can make a rattle (between two yoghurt pots stuck together, for example). Cooked it can be threaded on string. (Popcorn snacks are one of the easiest to make, and to vacuum up afterwards.)

Baked potatoes: there are lots of things to do with potatoes – shapes, prints, etc. – and children can also be involved in mixing the scooped-out contents of cooked potatoes with cheese, cottage cheese, etc., and restuffing the skins.

There can be some unexpected spin-offs from the child's interest in foods. Children often bring home the ideas they pick up during their day-care, and so start to change the activities, and diets, that they and their family have at home. In one example, a child insisted his mother get wholemeal bread from now on, something the family had not eaten before. The boy even insisted he try to make bread at home. In another example, a child wanted some fresh fruit – satsumas, which the mother had not offered him before – instead of his usual packet pudding. It is at times like these that the whole effort seems worthwhile!

Racism and food

Many day-care centres have a racially and culturally mixed group of children. Even those that don't might want to provide their children with experiences of other cultures to prepare them for later life. Yet how many such day-care facilities take care to provide multi-ethnic menus?

The use of 'British' food day after day can undermine the children's respect for other types of food and sorts of cuisine. If they themselves are from a black or ethnic minority background with its own traditional cuisine then the child's respect for its own culture may be undermined. This may be despite the fact that many traditional foods and cuisines that have come to Britain from other parts of the world may actually be nutritionally better than typical 'British' diets.

Furthermore, many things that are considered British are

actually imported ideas from elsewhere. Potatoes originally came from the Andes. Turkeys came from North America. Cauliflowers come from the orient and rhubarb came from Russia. These foods were hardly known in Britain just a dozen generations ago. Ice cream came from China by way of Arabia and Italy. Pizza, spaghetti, popcorn, hamburgers, baked beans – all these are recent imports into our diet.

Ideas for making changes can be found all around. Some catering staff will have ideas of their own, and skills which have rarely been shown. Parents and relatives of the children may be encouraged to participate in making changes and bringing in ideas from their homes. Sometimes staff might feel unskilled, or inhibited, about making changes and need to be encouraged. If it is a matter of not having the right skills and understanding, then sometimes the appropriate parents or relatives can be asked to participate in making changes – they can come and give a demonstration of how things are done at home, and can provide recipes, show how utensils are used, what spices are included and how the food should be served.

Festivals and celebrations can make the changes into a special occasion: Caribbean Week could be organised around carnival time, for example, or a special Far Eastern day at Chinese New Year. These are excellent means of bringing in parents and relatives to get them more involved, contributing their ideas and experiences and learning about the day-care centre at the same time. There is one danger though: one nursery put on a Jamaican Week for the many children whose families had come from Jamaica. This was great – except that for the rest of the year the word Jamaica was hardly ever mentioned, and Jamaican culture was never explored. So in making a special occasion it is important to remember that the cultural needs continue throughout the rest of the year.

Here are some of the festivals and special occasions celebrated by various groups of people, which might make a focus for cultural learning activities among young children, and which can help to bring parents and relatives into the day-care centre. Special occasions are not, of course, substitutes for ensuring that there is multicultural respect every day of the year

(continues)

Rastafarian New Year (7 January)

Chinese New Year (late January or early February)

Tu b'Shevat (Jewish new year for trees, late January or early February)

Lohri (Hindu festival marking the end of winter, during January)

Setsuban (Japanese bean-scattering ceremony, 3 February)

Carnival (Latin American and Caribbean festival, often linked to Shrove Tuesday, in February or early March)

Holi (Hindu spring festival, during February or March)

Ching Ming (Chinese festival of light, usually during March)

Naw-Ruz (Baha'i New Year, 21 March)

Ploughing Festival (Buddhist festival a week before *Wesak*)

Jamshedi Noruz (Fasli calendar new year, 21 March)

Wesak (Buddhist festival, first day of full moon in May)

Shavout (Jewish Feast of Weeks, late May, early June)

Obon (Japanese festival around 15 July)

Farvardigan (Shahenshai occasion, ten days before *No Ruz*)

No Ruz (Shahenshai new year, around the end of August)

Rosh Hoshanah (Jewish new year, usually September)

Chung-Yang (Chinese kite festival, late September or early October)

Dussehra (ten-day Hindu celebration, usually during October)

Divali (Hindu new year festival, during October or November)

Shichi-go-san (Japanese festival for boys of 7, girls of 5, boys of 3, 15 November)

Ramadan (Muslim month for fasting, moves earlier each solar year: due to start early April 1989, late March 1990, mid-March 1991, early March 1992, etc.)

Id al Fitr (Muslim festival, at the end of *Ramadan*)

Al Hijrah (Muslim new year, fourteen weeks after *Id al Fitr*)

Ashura (Muslim two-day fast, ten days after *Al Hijrah*)

These are just some of the possibilities. If you include all the National Days celebrated in various countries around the world then there could be a party virtually every day! But remember there is no substitute for asking around and finding out what is happening locally.

Serving and eating food can differ between cultures and this, too, needs exploring and encouraging. In some cultures only the right hand is used for eating, and it is carefully washed before and after each meal. In others, chopsticks may be used. Mouths are often rinsed out after eating. These habits can be more hygienic than common practices in Britain, yet they might be given little recognition and even laughed at – further undermining the children's attitudes and respect for their own and other people's backgrounds.

The attitudes of staff and other adults present can be crucial. Giving the children a variety of foods while not eating it oneself can make the children anxious about the food and its 'difference', and subtly destroy all the work that has been done. Everyone involved in making changes towards more multicultural initiatives needs to know why they are doing it, and want to participate.

Besides the food and the festivities, some of the play-time activities need to be looked at. Most play areas have a play-house of some description. How many of these are equipped with cooking and eating utensils from the different cultures? Are there pictures of fruit and vegetables, for example, on the wall or in books – and do these represent what the children actually experience, at home or in the day-care centre?

Positive reinforcement of children's own and each others' backgrounds can be given to children in a number of ways, especially by showing that the way they live at home is recognised and supported in the day-care centre, centre. In the same way, the changes made at the day-care centre, and the attitudes and expectations of the staff, can have repercussions on the parents and relatives.

The involvement of parents in nursery activities is valuable, but it is difficult for many working parents to arrange. At a conference run by the National Committee on Racism in Children's Books, in Birmingham, 1987, black parents expressed the view that they sometimes did not feel confident enough to make their view known at parents' meetings if they felt in a minority. They felt it important that the staff were committed, and showed their commitment to the children by eating the same food, for example. But in the end, staff attitudes were, the conference felt, more important than making changes to the food because if staff were not enthusiastic then nothing else would overcome this. Among the various strategies recommended at the conference was the suggestion that nursery nurse courses and playgroup staff training should include both instruction on basic nutrition and diets on the one hand, and training in the needs and preferences of various cultures in Britain in relation to what they eat: in other words, training on food and racism. Food can be potentially an area for racism and cultural domination, or alternatively it can be an area for multicultural learning and anti-racist activity, for black and white children alike.

Taste Tables – a food-related version of Activity Tables – have been tried in several nurseries and found to be successful. The idea is to offer to children (and perhaps their parents, too) an opportunity to try out things they may never have met before. This means giving them a chance to explore and experience different tastes and textures, different fruits and vegetables, foods from different cultures and so forth, *without feeling themselves to be under the sort of pressure that would happen at meal-time.*

A Taste Table could be small and limited: different breads, or different cheeses, for example. Or it could be more ambitious: foods from the Caribbean or from South-East Asia, for example. They can be related foods: everything in season in a particular country, say, or a selection of dips made from soya tofu. Different staple foods can be compared: e.g. plantain, yam, cassava, maize meal, rice flour, sorghum, dahl and couscous.

Here is one nursery's ambitious Taste Table spread, presented on a special occasion. Letters had been circulated to the children's families, and the Taste Table was designed to interest parents as much as children:

- Various cheeses, including vegetarian and goat's cheese
- Halva (ground sesame seeds with honey and nuts)
- Trail mix, and Tropical mix
- Bombay mix (spicy)
- Fresh crab and fresh prawns
- Bean curd mixed with ginger and soya sauce

(continues)

- Humus, taramasalata and chilli dips
- Raw vegetable sticks, for the dips
- Banana bread
- Chilean Christmas bread
- Seven different salamis and sausages
- Fruits: Mango, Hunza, Sharron fruit
- Onion Bhaji
- Falafil (made from chick-peas)
- Fresh and tinned lychees, to compare

Whenever possible, the food can be accompanied by details about what it is and where it originally came from. People will ask the name of the dish or the fruit, how it is prepared, how it is normally eaten, where it can be bought, and what the recipe is. In many cases it may be wise to involve some parents beforehand, perhaps even getting them to do it themselves.

Food means work, and costs money

Preparing even a simple snack takes time. Preparing a full meal for a nursery takes a lot of time, and may be a paid job for one or two catering staff. But if the recommendations for healthier diets mean moving away from packaged and processed foods and towards more fresh ingredients, are we making more work for the staff responsible? For a start, the total time needed may not actually add up to a great deal more than before. But it might well need greater skill on the cook's part. This can be a positive bonus. In one Southwark nursery, where more fresh food is now being used, the cook is very enthusiastic. 'At last', she says 'I am doing something interesting using skills that I forgot I had.'

The sorts of changes she has made are largely in the methods she uses: much less roasting and deep-frying, much more baking and boiling, steaming and stir-frying. In some instances, she has cut back on her cooking time: fruit and vegetables are simply cut and presented in an attractive way, with little more preparation needed than that. Raw fruit takes no more time than the old instant whips, and is actually simpler than blancmange or custard.

Salads are easy too. And, as we discussed earlier, the children might want to be involved in making some of these menu items.

There may also be less waste. The children at one nursery now serve themselves from bowls, taking what they feel they want. And even if there is food left in the bowls, if this is fresh it can be used again in a cooked meal the following day. There isn't much you can do with left-over instant whip, but plenty you can do with apples and bananas.

The cook at this nursery has found that there is more scope to put in spices and flavours to suit the children's taste, rather than accept what the manufacturer put in the ready-to-eat package. So again there is less likelihood of waste, and greater opportunity to try a variety of different dishes from various cultures. From the cook's point of view life has become more interesting. The same is true for the children. And from the social services end, the budget is actually little changed from before: although some fresh foods cost more than their processed counterparts, other expensive foods have been dropped altogether and replaced with less costly, but just as healthy alternatives.

Fresh fruit out of season costs more than a canned version of the same fruit. But dahl and chappatis are cheaper than burgers and chips, and very nutritious too. Spaghetti hoops from a tin may be less trouble than fresh pasta and fresh sauce. But a few minutes of steaming vegetables may be less trouble, and cheaper, than an hour roasting. Apple 'faces' with dried fruit is cheaper and easier than suet pudding, and needs no cooking at all.

All in all the total costs need not alter a great deal. The experiences of some larger institutions (such as NHS hospitals) have shown that changing to a healthier diet can be just as cheap and more cost-effective, with less waste or overprovision. People may claim that going over to a healthier diet is expensive for an institution like a nursery, but often this is based on the impressions given by health food shops, where even the simplest item can seem overpriced. Let the person who makes such a claim show why they think it will happen, and even if it turns out that they may be right, we have to ask 'what are the costs of *not* making the diet healthier?' 'What do we want for our children?'

A Case History

This is the diary of one nursery in Lancashire that wanted to cut out some of the processed foods and additives, and bring in more fresh food: 'Food that didn't need lists of ingredients'.

June We have fifteen children referred to us as hyperactive, and the high incidence of diarrhoea was giving cause for concern.

The staff made some enquiries to see whether the children were eating the right sort of food. We decided to cut down on sugar and to include more fresh food. We wanted to reduce the food termed 'junk' and try and cut out colourings, additives and preservatives.

July We requested from our supplies officer certain changes in our orders:
- Wholemeal bread
- Wholemeal flour
- Fresh orange juice
- Pure vegetable fat
- Sugar-free jam
- Natural breakfast cereals

The request was granted, and we started to introduce these foods at breakfast and tea-time.

August We started to introduce more wholefood items, gradually, and to cut back on red meats. The menus were planned to include a meat-free week once every month.

September We asked for a breakdown of the daily cost of food per child, which turned out (at 65 pence) to be well within the limits compared with other, similar nurseries.

The high rate of diarrhoea will be monitored as we gradually change over to more wholefoods.

(continues)

October We decided to arrange a parents evening to explain the new policies on food, and test their reaction to the idea of a completely wholefood diet. We contacted a nutritionist who agreed to speak at the evening.

November We presented a report to our social services meeting of officers and senior management. Many questions were asked, and we agreed to monitor the situation and report back in February.

The parents evening was a great success. Nearly three-quarters of all the parents came, sixty-three people, and the nutritionist's talk stimulated a lot of discussion, which went on for weeks. As a result we decided to introduce a completely wholefood diet starting in January.

January We had one case of diarrhoea, on 14 January, but this was a child who had not attended nursery since before Christmas.

In conjunction with the introduction of the wholefood diet, we have started several projects to develop the children's awareness of food. We hope that the children, parents and staff, as well as the general public, will all help to learn about food and start to question the type of foods presently being manufactured, and promoted through advertising campaigns often aimed specifically at children.

signed: Officer in Charge and Deputy Officer in Charge.

In a later report, the management identified three key elements to the success of this project: gradual changes in the menu; the food awareness projects; and the involvement of the parents. It was also noted that there was little difficulty getting the children to accept the changes: 'Maybe it is time we destroyed the myth that left to their own devices children chose "junk" food.'

The case history is not taken from a nursery serving middle-class 'motivated' parents. Of the children in this nursery, 80 per cent were children with 'special needs' from socially deprived backgrounds. The success of the project was reflected in the enthusiasm of the children and staff, along with parents, social workers, health visitors and the general public (through a project at the local library) all being drawn in.

Additives at the nursery

If there is one thing parents are most anxious about, it is additives. Parents are worried about reports of ill health linked to additives, and although they can take care about what they feed their children at home, they do not have the same control over what their children get when they are looked after in day-care centres. So they come to the staff, and ask whether there are any additives in what their little one is being given to eat.

In fact, only a few children are likely to be really intolerant of additives, and come out with symptoms like asthma or hyper-activity. But even if it is only one in several thousand who might react like this it is worth being concerned – why add to the number of risks they are already exposed to? Furthermore, some additives may have long-term effects which are not fully under-stood. So a playgroup or nursery that wants to take action on additives needs to sit and have a think.

Generally, there are two things a nursery could do. Either they can make a special case of the children whose parents are worried, and make sure that those children are not served with anything that might put them at risk. Sometimes this ends up like a punishment, with the at-risk child not allowed to have what the other children are all enjoying. The second option is to change the diet for everyone, so that nobody is put at risk. This may sound drastic, but actually it is not so difficult. The goals are these:

- avoid additives by using fresh food
- eliminate all the additive-rich foods that you reasonably can
- cut back on the additive-rich foods that you do need to use
- look for alternatives with fewer or no alternatives

Many of the changes that are being recommended nowadays for eating more healthily – cutting back on highly processed foods and offering more fresh foods and 'whole' foods – will at the same time remove many of the sources of unwanted additives from the menu. Offering fresh orange juice – even the packets of orange as long as they are pure – with nothing added, instead of orange squash, will immediately cut all the colourings, added sugars, bits of orange skin and other undesirables, including the additives. Swapping fruit or vegetables for biscuits at snack time will cut out all the fats and sugars, and the added preservatives and anti-oxidants, colourings and added flavourings.

The sorts of questions that need to be asked are: 'Can we find economical alternatives to sweet biscuits and orange squash?' Many nurseries and playgroups are moving towards healthier foods, with fruit, fruit juices, sandwiches and milk being suggested instead. A few places are now looking at ways of turning these changes to their advantage by using them as part of the day's activities. For example, they buy an unusual fruit – a melon, say – and make a special show about where it came from, how it is opened, slicing it up, sharing it out and using the seeds afterwards. And one nursery in Peckham has declared itself to be *An Additive-free Zone*!

LEAVING NURSERY

Making the changes will not come overnight, and for the children's stomach's sake it is better if they are not made overnight – a sudden introduction to large doses of fibre, such as changing from refined 'white' flour to wholegrains and fruit and vegetables, can lead to upset stomachs, cramps and wind. The changes should be brought about gradually, over weeks rather than days. But the results in the long term will be worthwhile. The child will develop habits of eating which will stand them in good stead all their lives ... if nothing comes along to destroy these good habits.

Which is where we come to school. Even the best of children may be tempted by some of the worst that schools can offer. All the good work and enthusiasm can be lost in just a few weeks when poor little Johnny leaves day-care and starts at Reception Class, with his name down for school dinner. This is not to cast aspersions at the well-intentioned and honourable catering staff in schools. It is to remind us, though, that schools provide food for a growing child for at least ten of the most important years of their life from a health point of view. Damage done at this age will not be easily repaired, and habits learnt will be hard to break later. We have a responsibility to see that school dinners are as good as they can be, following the latest accepted advice on healthy, sound nutrition, caring for those that most need to be offered the best that can be given. Is this what they get?

Unfortunately not. For many children, school is where the opportunities for healthy eating are lost, put second to the needs of the education authorities to meet their budgets, which are set, in turn, by central government. A lot of politics falls eventually on the school dinner plate.

SCHOOL MEALS

You might think that school was just the place for children to learn about healthy eating. But, unfortunately, since the 1980 Education Act removed the duty of schools to meet certain nutritional standards, many schools have started to sell food which they can count on to sell well, rather than food which most nutritionists would think of as healthy.

A government survey in 1984 investigating the foods older school children were eating found that large quantities of foods like crisps, chips and biscuits were being consumed. Some children had such poor diets that they were going seriously short of essential vitamins and minerals. But now that the free school meal provision has been abolished for an estimated half a million children (all those previously eligible under Family Income Supplement, now Family Credit), even the poorest families will start wondering if they should forget school meals and try to provide their children with food themselves, or give them the money to buy food out of school.

Only those children who were previously entitled to free school meals under Supplementary Benefit (now Income Support) will still be entitled to receive something – and that something can be fairly meagre. One local authority is reported to give, as a free meal, a packed lunch consisting of a savoury sandwich, a flapjack and a handful of raisins.

The trend is away from school meals, and if nothing is done to reverse this, the whole service may gradually become a historical memory, a dead fossil from the mid twentieth century. Fortunately, school meals are still a central part of the daily nutrition for the majority of school-children and they can, and in many places still do, make an important contribution to the nourishment of the children they serve, and hence the growth and development of the next generation. Indeed, some education authorities are creating attractive services with high standards. These good examples need to be encouraged. Where the system is falling short of good standards it needs to be criticised, and the people who can do this most effectively are the children and their parents as the consumers.

Recent history

In 1975, what many authorities had been doing voluntarily became official guidance: the school meal was required to offer children at least one-third of their daily nutritional needs. Less than this, and the local authority would infringe the guidelines.

Then, just five years later, the 1980 Education Act removed that requirement, and a local authority could offer whatever it liked – cola and boiled sweets, or just a packet of crisps, if they wished. Over the next few years, school meals services were – and continue to be – squeezed by cash limits on their spending, and by the threat of being opened to private tendering, so the pressure was to find ways of providing food that parents wouldn't object to, that children would accept, that did not cost a great deal, and that needed the minimum of staff. Fast food-style canteens were the answer tried by some local authorities, with an emphasis on foods which are advertised and promoted to children on TV and in magazines. Crisps, chips, soft drinks and sugary foods were put on offer, and eaten up by hungry children.

The squeeze was tightened further in 1984, when the Treasury – which had been subsidising much of the cost of meals provided by local authorities – said it was cutting its contribution by a third, from £415m in 1984/85 down to £280m in 1986/87. Services across the country felt the pinch badly. The prices charged to children who did not get free meals rose substantially, and as a result the numbers taking dinner at school fell. Many children took packed lunches from home, or else went to buy snacks at local shops.

Then legislation in 1988 removed the right to have free school meals for all children in families eligible for Family Income Supplement (Family Credit). This amounted to an estimated half a million children from lower income families on low earnings. Families who were on Supplementary Benefit (now Income

Support) were to remain entitled to free school meals, but the withdrawal of free school meals from Family Credit children will still affect about half of the very children most in need of adequate nourishment.

At the same time, the number of jobs in school meals services has been cut. Traditionally, these workers have usually been part-time, and most of them are women, and it is they who are the main target for cost-cutting. Since the introduction of cafeteria-style catering in schools, an estimated 50,000 jobs have been cut, and even for those still in work, pay and entitlements have been cut. It is not surprising if workers feel demoralised and under attack, rather than valued for the useful work they do.

Struggling for better meals

We looked at the sort of food served up as 'fast' or convenient food in an earlier part of this book. The sort served up in schools is likely to be much the same as that found in your average take-away or fast food outlet. These foods are high in fat, sugar and salt, and low in fibre. The cooking methods are likely to involve deep-fat frying, double-cooking and reheating – all of them destroying valuable nutrients and adding extra, unnecessary calories.

This doesn't mean that children have to give up what they appear to be enjoying so much – although many children would change to healthier food if it was available. It does mean, for all children, a matter of getting a balance. Fatty items should be less dominant on the plate, while fresh fruits and vegetables, and the pulses, and whole grain foods should feature more often.

School caterers need to be encouraged to provide meals based on more health-conscious recipes: aiming to make them lower in fat, sugar and salt, and higher in fibre. And they will need to ensure that their menus are acceptable to children with particular dietary requirements and offer a range of cultural choices.

Here are some practical suggestions that can be put to the school catering service. They do not cover the full range of possibilities that might be needed, but provide a starting point for parents and teachers, children and catering staff to get discussing what they want and how they are going to get it. In the later parts of this book we will outline the overall dietary advice for younger children on which these suggestions here are made. And in the next section, Telling Them What We Want, we shall give some suggestions about who you should talk to, or write to, to get something done.

IDEAS FOR MAKING SCHOOL MEALS BETTER

Cutting fatty foods

- Alternatives to fatty foods should be available at every meal. One low-fat main course and one low-fat dessert should be available every day. Crisps should be the fat-reduced variety, and alternatives like nuts and raisins should be available. Boiled, mashed or jacket potatoes should be available besides chips.
- Meat products should be low-fat if possible, and should be grilled or baked rather than fried. Some local education authorities have asked their suppliers to order low-fat sausages and burgers.
- Chips should be cut larger, should not be precooked, and should be cooked quickly in hot fat, and then drained on kitchen paper. Prefried chips should be avoided.
- Milk used for sauces, custards and puddings could be skimmed or semi-skimmed.
- Cheese used in cooking, salads and sandwiches can be the low-fat variety.

Cutting sugary foods

- Yoghurts with no added sugar should be available.
- Fruit should be offered in place of sweet desserts.
- Water should be freely available with every meal. There should be no need for children to buy soft drinks if they do not want to.
- Milkshakes could be made with fresh fruit instead of sweet mixes.

Cutting salt

- Table salt can be kept with other condiments at one place in the dining room, rather than put on every table.
- Cooking salt should be kept to minimum, and not used at all in salty dishes, such as those with cheese or bacon in them.

Boosting fibre-rich foods

- Salads could be provided at a self-service bar, preferably located within easy reach of small children, and located at the beginning of the serving area.
- Wholemeal bread should be provided and put at the front of the counter.
- Fruit should always be available at every meal.
- Sandwiches should be made with large rolls and baps containing some protein-rich food as well as salad vegetables. Brown and wholemeal breads should dominate.
- Vegetables should be fresh and served as soon as possible after cooking. They should have been steamed or cooked in only a little water, without any added salt or bicarbonate of soda.

It is not much point making these changes if children don't realise they are happening, and don't understand what they can choose from. It is just as important to keep children well informed as it is to make these changes in the first place.

These principles of healthy eating can be taught at school, and can make a valuable addition to any core curriculum being developed for schools generally. This doesn't just mean putting in a few words about healthy diets into a Home Economics or Domestic Science course. It means putting up posters and doing projects as part of all children's education at various ages throughout their school years.

Who Educates the Children?

Doing school projects on food is hardly a new idea. Food manufacturers have been approaching schools and providing them with free, or subsidised, 'information packs' for teachers to use with a class.

According to *Business International* magazine, children are a desirable advertising target because of their proven ability to influence adult purchasing behaviour. The child market is attractive to corporations that sell food, such as breakfast cereals and fast food. To woo the child, they have developed sophisticated cartoon characters and phantasy people – such as Tony the Tiger (Kellogg's Frosties) and Ronald McDonald (McDonald's). According to one survey in America, children could recall, and *said they preferred*, corporate characters such as Tony the Tiger and Ronald McDonald over grandpa, daddy or the local priest.

The large food companies are keen to get into schools, and have their names spread around by the teachers in classrooms. Here is a list of just some of the companies who have distributed 'project packs' and other forms of material like booklets, posters and videos into the schools of Britain:

All About Bread (*Allinson*)
Use Your Loaf (*Allinson*)
Energy for Fitness (*Allinson*)
The Whole Bread Story (*Allinson*)
Nutrition for Life (*Allinson and Help the Aged*)
Healthy Eating Investigations (*Boots*)
Eating Wisely, Eating Well (*British Nutrition Foundation and Roche Products*)
Diet and Heart Disease (*Flora*)
You Are What You Eat (*Flour Advisory Bureau*)
Nutrition in Action (*Heinz*)
Grains are Great Foods (*Kellogg*)
Good Food Your Choice (*Kellogg*)
Wheel of Food and Good Health (*Milk Marketing Board*)
Taste Invaders (*Milk Marketing Board*)
The Food Store (*Snack Nut and Crisp Manufacturers Association*)
Plant Sugars and Man (*Sugar Bureau*)
Nutrition Without Tears (*Sugar Bureau*)

Making changes

It is not all doom and gloom. Some local authorities have made a real effort to improve their meals, and to improve the information children receive about what they eat. For example, there are several menu-labelling schemes around the country, which might work for your school. In Surrey, the schools have a 'traffic light' system in the cafeterias. The food is marked with a traffic light indicating:

RED: Stop and Think, before you eat too many of these foods (for foods high in fat, sugar and salt)

GREEN: Go, go go! These are the Good Guys, eat plenty of them (for foods high in fibre)

AMBER: Go Carefully, eat these foods in moderation (for the rest)

Surrey also gives a special promotion to healthy foods such as jacket potatoes with tasty fillings. They have found that their children now eat 40 per cent fewer chips than before and 1100 per cent more jacket potatoes!

Another example comes from North Yorkshire. Children in schools there have been introduced to 'Herbie', the carrot who pops up on the menu to indicate the healthy choices. A walking, talking, life-size Herbie visits schools and talks to children about healthy eating.

North Yorkshire has also tried changing the atmosphere in school canteens, making them more attractive to children without sacrificing food quality. Pop music and modern decor has been introduced, and food is served from 'Hissing Sid's Grill' or 'Captain Beaky's Salad Bar'. At a school in Fulford the meals are served in a brightly coloured Burger Bar-style setting, with coloured furniture and smart fittings. It doesn't actually sell burgers, but instead offers jacket potatoes with fillings, cold meats, salads, soup, yoghurt, and wholemeal bread. It all helps to turn good food into fun food.

In Haringey, North London, the menu has been gradually changing over the years. New items are introduced with an organised 'taste-in' at school, open to parents and children. Here they test the proposed new dish and give their verdict, before it appears on the school menu.

At Millfields School in Bromsgrove, parents and children are invited to a Good Food Day Breakfast, where they can eat crusty wholemeal bread, sugar-free muesli and fruit.

Many other authorities have been trying out the changes towards better food that the parents have been asking for. The school meals service in Avon has been developing new menus and recipes, and schools in Gloucester have been cutting down on the fats and sugars and increasing the wholemeal flour in their pies and crumbles. Inner London schools have adapted painlessly to low-sugar baked beans and low-fat sausages with some of the additives removed.

These are examples from around the country. If they can do it – if they can provide good, healthy food at reasonable prices in attractive surroundings – then why can't your school meals service? Ask them. Ask why your school can't do the same.

In the next section we include some advice about who to approach at your school, and how to handle what they say in reply.

.. AND THEN WE WENT AND HAD SOME *BURGERS* AND THIS MAN GAVE ME A *HAT* AND DO YOU KNOW WHAT HE GAVE ONE TO MY *TEDDY* AS WELL IT'S MY **FAVOURITE** PLACE SOME-TIMES MUMMY MAKES BEEF-BURGERS FOR TEA BUT THEY'RE **NOT THE SAME!**

At four years old Molly's greatest treat
Is Mechanically Recovered Meat
Emulsified and stabilised,
Neutralised and well disguised
Re-formed into 'steaks' and 'burgerettes'
Enhanced with various glutamates,
Added water, colour, pure pig fat ...
Why waste putting any lean beef in that?

6 Making a Fuss

TELLING THEM WHAT *WE* WANT

A keen health advocate may try to convince us that anything processed is junk, but those of us with jobs, with children, or with little time or enthusiasm to cook know better. We know our children aren't going to die from eating the occasional tinned breakfast purée, packet beef and vegetable dinner, sweetened corn flakes or a burger and fries supper. At the same time, we know that such food does not rate highly on the health scales. And we may not be too pleased by the way some of the companies advertise their products to children and even get into the school classrooms.

But what can we do? We can act as individuals, making individual choice. Much of this book is devoted to giving the information that can help you make these choices between products. Slowly, the choice of items will get reflected in company sales sheets, and they will start to take notice. But voting with our purse or wallet is a very slow and inefficient way of communicating with the senior decision-makers in the larger companies and government ministries, the faceless few who make the decisions affecting the day-to-day content of what we are sold and what we could be sold.

Better by far if we could speak to them directly. Producing this book is one means, of course, as it might eventually get onto the shelves of the company libraries and ministry research departments. But we need to do more than this if we are to have the effect we need.

First, we need to sort our exactly what we are suggesting and to whom we are suggesting it. We can construct a list of things we want to see changed – perhaps a list like the Charter at the end of this book. We need to make it clear that we are not happy with some of the present practices, and that we want to see changes. After all, our children have a right to good quality foods, made to high standards. And the people who can defend their interests are, finally, us.

It may seem pointless to write letters and make telephone calls, but in fact it is not. A company that does not want to change and develop may well feel defensive about its producers, but a company that has an eye to the future all the time will actually welcome criticism and complaints, for it is from these that they can spot new markets and the potential for new products. Consumers' voices are the source of many a good idea for company bosses, and in this sense we have to feed them with what we want them to feed to us.

We believe writing letters can have an influence, especially if copies are sent to legislators and consumer groups at the same time. We have included some addresses for doing this in the last part of this chapter.

GO BACK TO THE SHOP

The food industry – especially the retailers – are continually competing for your custom. They don't want to lose you as a shopper, and more importantly, they want to know what the next trend is going to be. So they need to hear what you have to say, no matter how uncomfortable it may be for them.

You might, of course, know more about what you are complaining of, or demanding, than your local grocery store. They might well feel uncomfortable, and try giving you a non-answer, like 'I'm sorry madam, this is how the product comes from our suppliers.' This isn't much use to you. You have to persist and explain why the supplier should be told of your dissatisfaction, or why the grocery should use a different supplier. If you have taken the trouble to get your facts right, you may find that you know more about what you are talking about than the shop manager.

Even your local supermarket manager may not know what you are talking about, but he or she will have the sense, usually, to realise that what you have to say could mean more sales and even good publicity if he or she acts upon it. They may do nothing themselves, but they would be fools not to let their regional manager know, who might well bring it up at the next sales and products meeting. 'Consumer resistance to such-and-such a product', they mention, or 'Complaints about so-and-so company – some mothers are saying they won't stand for it.'

WRITE TO THE COMPANY

Sometimes it's quicker to write straight to the customer relations departments of the companies, spelling out your views and making your suggestions. The address should be printed on every packet. Write to that address, addressing the letter to their *customer relations* or *customer enquiry* departments. If you want to mention a specific product, then try to indicate exactly which product you mean: its name, the size and any codes you can see on the pack. It may also help them to identify the product if you indicate where and when you bought it.

Companies will usually respond to your letters. They are unlikely to put them in the bin without a second thought. And two or three such letters in a week will make them take a lot of notice. If you really want to make them sympathetic, tell them about some examples of things you like. If they or a competitor are doing something which you approve of, put that in your letter.

So, in summary, if you are unhappy or dissatisfied with a product, and you want to tell the company concerned to get the product changed, then write to them. If you can,

- identify the product as clearly as possible
- say what you are unhappy about
- make suggestions for changes
- give examples of better products
- get other people to write, too
- send copies of your letter to other relevant people, such as your local Trading Standards Office (at your local authority) and the shop where you bought the product, and perhaps to a consumers' organisation, and the media, too.

SOMETHING IS SERIOUSLY WRONG

If you feel you have a complaint about a product which may actually be breaking the law, or should certainly have something done about it fast – like a piece of glass in the purée, or a misleading label which could be dangerous – then get some professional help. The people to turn to in such cases are to be found in your local authority: the Environmental Health and Trading Standards Departments.

Each local authority will organise its consumer services differently, and so you may find that environmental health officers will deal with both problems we gave as examples, or trading standards officers, or they may split the problems with environmental health dealing with food quality, and trading standards dealing with labelling. Some local authorities have combined the two into one department, called Consumer Protection or Public Protection. Don't worry. How they divide their duties is up to them, and as far as you are concerned you have a legitimate complaint for them to deal with.

These same departments are also able to offer advice and information on the law and how you can use it. They have pamphlets and guides on how you can make complaints. They are also in a position to collect evidence locally, so they may tell you that you are not the first to make your complaint.

If you don't feel satisfied with the service you get from the officers in these departments then you may want to take the issue one step higher. Local authority departments are answerable to local councillors – your locally elected politicians who run the Town Hall or County Hall including these departments. The councillors form groups or committees to oversee these departments, so you may want to find out who is the chair of the Environmental Health Committee, for example, or Public Protection Committee. Again, each local authority has its own way of organising committees. If they seem too baffling, then go and see your own local councillors at their regular surgery if they hold one, or go to your nearest advice centre.

IS THE AUTHORITY ITSELF TO BLAME?

Of course, when it comes to school dinners, or even to nursery snacks, it may turn out that you have to make your views known to the local authority itself, as they are responsible for the schools and nurseries they run.

With nurseries and playgroups, there are two possibilities. The nursery or playgroup concerned may be actually run by the local authority social services department: these are *maintained* day-care facilities for under 5s. Or they may be independent nurseries and playgroups, which still are supposed to be *registered* with the social services department, and may actually receive a grant from that department. So you need to check out which of the situations applies.

If they are registered facilities, then they will have their own management structure, and you will have to work at getting yourself heard by that management. If they don't give you the satisfaction you feel you deserve, then you can complain about them to the social services department, whose job is to ensure that the nursery or playgroup comes up to standard. If it is falling below standards then social services will take up your grievance and start to insist that changes are made. If it does not fall below standards then of course it could be that the standards are too low – in which case you need to work on changing the social services' policies on registering playgroups and nurseries generally.

Maintained nurseries and playgroups are part of social services' own provision for the needs of under 5s. To make changes you need to work through social service department officers responsible for under 5s, starting with the officer-in-charge at the nursery itself.

If it still turns out that social services' policies are not what you feel is right, then you need to get the policies changed. Just as with the Environmental Health and Trading Standards departments, the social services staff are answerable to your local councillors, and their Social Services Committee. So, again, it would be to the councillors on that committee, or else your own local councillors, that you need to turn.

With schools, the situation is similar, and there are more possible sources of help that you can turn to. For example, your school may have a *parent-teacher association* (PTA) where the issue can be raised, and where other parents or relatives can express their views and perhaps give you encouragement.

The PTA is a fairly informal meeting. If you need to get more formal, then it may be useful to ask to put your case to a meeting of the *school governors*. These have parent-representatives on them, and it might be valuable to have a chat with one of these parent-governors first. The names of the parent-governors, and the dates for their meetings, can usually be given to you at the school office or head teacher's office. The school governors may not be able to do anything themselves, as they do not have direct responsibility for the meals. But they can decide to support your proposals and lend their weight to your campaign, which might make the meals service more likely to listen to you.

It may also be worth talking to the *head teacher*, or deputy head, about your feelings. Although they are not directly responsible for the school meals services, they do have a responsibility for the well-being of all the children, and may also have some experience of handling the meals staff and catering officers who provide the meals. If there is a school tuck-shop, and you have feelings about what the tuck-shop sells, then again you might want to start by talking to the head, who can direct you to the people running the tuck shop.

School *meals staff* can be talked to about your concerns. The cooks and assistants will not, by and large, be the ones responsible for actually deciding what is on the menu and where the supplies come from. But they will be the ones who would have to implement any major changes, and this may mean they will have to learn new skills and change routines. It is worth making sure that your ideas are greeted sympathetically by the catering staff, and that they don't feel threatened by what you are proposing. Too many jobs have been lost in the name of 'improvements' for them to feel happy about making any more changes. One person who can help you through this sticky area is the local *trade union* representative – who is likely to be a member of either the National Union of Public Employees (NUPE) or the General, Municipal, Boilermakers and Allied Workers Union (now simply called GMB). The staff can be asked who their shop steward or local official is, or you can find out from the union's local offices – see the phone book.

In charge of the kitchen staff are the *catering managers*, who are part of the education authority's management structure. Their job is to oversee the delivery of the service, and this includes planning menus, ensuring the quality of the food is up to standard, and liaising with suppliers to get the products they want. There may be separate supplies officers responsible for ordering goods and arranging contracts, but ultimately the responsibility rests with the senior catering managers, or in some authorities, the *school meals organiser*. They are the ones who can answer questions about nutritional standards, menu labelling, the authority's present policies on, say, additives, the intended changes they are proposing for the meals service, the possibilities of changing suppliers and so forth. This is where your letters are likely to end up, but, of course, your letters will have more weight to them if you have the support of the PTA, the governors or the catering staff.

If you don't like the answers you get from the senior catering managers then you will have to take your ideas to the people they are answerable to – the *education authority*, which is run by the Education Committee of your local council. As with Environmental Health and Social Services Committees, you need to find a councillor who sits on the Education Committee, or else you should try your own local councillors at their evening surgery. Failing that, try contacting a councillor through the Town Hall, or through a local advice centre.

REINFORCEMENTS

It may help to make your case if you have some professional advice. A trick here is to get professionals from one authority to take your side against an authority where you are trying to have changes made. So you might turn to the NHS to get support about healthy eating, as a way of putting pressure on your local authority who are responsible for schools and nurseries.

Professionals are also useful if you need to arrange a meeting with a guest speaker, or you want to suggest that a class, or a library, or a nursery starts a project, such as 'healthy eating day'. There are several people whose job is to offer such help and give you the support you need.

First, when it comes to food, your local expert is the *district dietitian*. Dietitians can be found working at your local District Hospital, and in some dietetics departments there are *community dietitians* whose main job is to work with groups in the community, rather than focusing on individual patients. So try and interest a community dietitian in your ideas, and perhaps invite them to your meetings, to be available to answer questions or even give a short talk.

The dietetics departments may also be able to provide posters, leaflets, video and other forms of display material, but more likely you will get a better response for such requests from your local *Health Education Department*. This department, too, can usually be found at your local District Hospital. The officers here have the prime task of promoting health education in the health district, and will have a range of materials available which could be of use to you. Try them. Again, you might like to invite a health education officer to your meetings, or into a classroom or nursery, or to help you mount an exhibition.

On the sugar and teeth front, you can also make good use of your local *District Dental Officer* who is also interested in promoting healthier eating, and will have leaflets and posters to offer and might be able to come to your meetings or talk to groups of children. They can be found through your local District Hospital or the Community Health Council.

Any of these three departments can also be contacted by first going to your local *Community Health Council* (CHC). The main function of this council is to represent the needs of the local community when it comes to making decisions about the health services. CHCs may also have leaflets and information sheets available for your use, and may be helpful and sympathetic in putting your case to the authorities you are dealing with. In the first case, contact the CHC Secretary, a full-time worker at the CHC – the number should be in the phone book.

RAISING THE STAKES

In the end, you may come up against the limits of what is presently possible. It may be that there is nothing you can do within the present law to achieve the changes you want.

To take your struggle further you will need to reach the people who make the laws and regulations which govern this society, who set the standards for what the food companies can and can't provide, and who say what the schools can and cannot do with their school dinner service. Part of our struggle, then, must be to put pressure on law-makers to get the regulations changed and to get resources put into the things that matter most.

This means putting pressure on local officials and local politicians, and on government ministries and Members of Parliament. It means working alone and with others so that your voice is heard and making sure that it cannot be ignored.

Journalist and author Geoffrey Cannon came across some facts which alarmed him: the extent to which Members of Parliament are linked to food industry interests. Of the 650 MPs in the House of Commons, 178 had some direct connection with food industry interests (this was in January 1987). The MPs may be consultants or advisers to food companies or food trade associations, they may be present or past directors or employees of food companies, or they may be owners of, or shareholders in, food companies. Over 50 per cent of Conservative MPs were found to have some food industry interests, while less than one in five Labour MPs had such interests.

Members of Parliament can be contacted through their local 'surgeries' or else through their Westminster offices. To find out who your MP is, when they hold surgeries, and how to reach them at other times, you can ring the House of Commons Library (tel. 01–219 4272). To contact an MP at the House of Commons, you can phone them at their offices there (tel. 01–219 3000 and ask to be put through to the MP you want).

Ministries are a different kettle of fish. The simplest approach is to write to the *Minister* of the ministry you think is most likely to be able to deal with your concern. The letter will be opened by somebody else, and almost certainly will be answered by somebody else. The minister is unlikely to see it. What the minister does look at, though, are letters from other MPs or from organisations which carry some clout. So if you can get them to send your letter on your behalf, which they will often do, you might receive a more detailed and considered reply. Even getting your local councillor or school governors to write the letter might ensure a better response.

Which ministry do you turn to? The main office responsible for food is the Ministry of Agriculture Fisheries and Food (MAFF), but to make things complicated, the policies on diet and health are not primarily their responsibility but are the responsibility of the Department of Health and Social Security (DHSS). Food companies might have to be complained about through the Department of Trade and Industry, and the concentration of power in large companies' hands should be referred to the Monopolies

Commission. Food worker issues might be dealt with by the Department of Employment, while some agricultural effects on the countryside are best dealt with by the Department of the Environment. Issues concerning foreign foodstuffs might have to go to the Foreign Office, or the Department of Transport (e.g. shipping) or Customs and Excise (importation). And now certain responsibilities are handled by the European Commission rather than the British government.

Expert advice is available to ministers and civil servants through a network of advisory committees. Food production, on the one hand, and the effects of consuming the food which is produced, on the other, are dealt with by different committees responsible to different ministries (MAFF and DHSS). Both ministries have a series of expert committees who advise them and help draft out the regulations which various authorities then try to enforce.

These expert committees are an interesting phenomenon. Without thinking too hard, we might assume that they consist mostly of senior, experienced scientists who can give the facts, a few consumer representatives to indicate what is wanted, some of the food inspectors and analysts who have to put the regulations into effect, plus some civil servants who can draft the legislation and turn theory into daily law.

If we thought this we would be wrong. For a start the members of government advisory committees are required to sign the Official Secrets Act. Anything they see or hear during their meetings cannot be repeated to anyone outside the room, by law. This makes it very difficult for anyone to represent consumer organisations, as they cannot report back on what happened in the committee. The committees may reach decisions, but these decisions are only recommendations – they may be ignored, overturned, amended or just delayed indefinitely. The members of the panel are selected by the civil servants, and it is worth taking a closer look at exactly who is selected.

In a thorough investigaton of twenty-seven official advisory committees over the period 1974–87, author Geoffrey Cannon identified whether there were any links with the interests of the food industry. The twenty-seven committees had room for a total of 370 seats, and of these an amazing 222 had food industry interests: 132 had been or were still actual employees of various food companies, 65 received funding from the food industry or else were consultants to various companies, 156 were involved in the British Nutrition Foundation, an industry-funded grouping set up in 1967 specifically to build links between industry interests and the government. Several committee members fell into more than one of these categories. And several committee members sat on more than one committee – on average they would each sit on two of the twenty-seven looked at in detail.

Who decides the main priorities for research into food? Several expert committees are involved in advising the government on the crucial topic concerning the spending of government money and effort investing food issues. These committees include:

ACARD – the Advisory Council on Applied Research and Development – reports to the Cabinet Office
Food Priorities Board – reports to MAFF
Food Processing Committee – advises Food Priorities Board
Food Quality Committee – advises Food Priorities Board
Food Safety Committee – advises Food Priorities Board

The chairperson of these powerful and influential committees was in every case a senior food industry person: Dr Douglas Georgala, head of research at Unilever; Sir Kenneth Durham, ex-chairman of Unilever; Dr Thomas Gorsuch, research director at Reckitt and Colman: Tony Good, ex-director of Grand Metropolitan and ex-chairman of Express Dairies; and Professor John Norris, research director at Cadbury Schweppes. In at least three of the committees there was no consumer representative at all.

In all, Geoffrey Cannon found twenty-seven companies represented on nineteen MAFF advisory committees, with one company alone (Unilever) having twelve people occupying twenty different committee seats. There were thirteen companies with interests in chocolates and sweets, cakes, biscuits, ice cream and soft drinks, and they occupied sixty of the committee seats on these nineteen advisory committees.

What sort of advice would these sixty people give? We can never know – it's a secret!

This complex web of powerful interests lies behind the organisation that you are writing to, when you write to a government ministry. Bureaucracies are not good at creating a sympathetic approach to the public, and may seem distant and unapproachable, and too good at stone-walling your requests. But do not despair, even stone walls can crumble if you keep on wearing away at them, and sometimes will just fall if you push at the right place.

STONE WALLS?

One problem with bureaucracies – especially those in large ministries – is that they are very skilled at writing letters which do not really help you. They start off by saying something like

'It can't be done'

to which you have to do one of two things. If you can prove it, you can say 'Yes it can' and have some examples ready. Or else you can challenge them: 'Why, exactly?' But obviously it helps if you do have some examples, if not from Britain then from other countries – Norway, say, where many colourings are banned, or Canada, where nutrition education is taught in schools.

Or else they may say

'We are already doing it'

to which you need to ask 'Really? Show me where.' You need to do this because it is sometimes the case that good policies have been adopted in principle but have not been put into practice. Perhaps there isn't actually an example they can show you, but they have said, on paper, that they are committed to doing what you are now suggesting. Get them to admit that *it hasn't actually happened yet*.

Or else they may say

'Children wouldn't eat it'

to which you need to argue that they will, and do. You need to make it clear that you are not asking for overnight changes if this would make something unpopular, but you are asking for modest steps to be taken, so that gradually the changes come about. Recipes may be gradually altered, certain ingredients eliminated, the atmosphere where it is offered improved (e.g. school canteens) or what you want should be offered alongside what is already available.

Or else they may say

'It is too expensive'

to which you need to argue that in fact it may well not be any more expensive, and even if it were it is money well spent. Switching to better food needn't cost any more – quite a lot of expensive processed products will be dropped in favour of cheaper but healthier products. Basing prices on an experience of a health food shop is a mistake – look instead in your largest supermarket and see what healthier foods cost there. Remember that eating unhealthy food is costing the NHS around £1 billion pounds each year as it is. Can we really afford *not* to improve everyone's diets, especially those of future generations?

Here are some more typical answers which you may be unfortunate enough to receive. But don't be put off by them. They are standard jargon and they will try it on if they can.

'We have never had any complaints about this.'

'Thank you for your letter. We shall look into the matter in due course ...'

'The issues you raise are not the concern of this Department.'

'The Ministry considered this issue last year as part of its review of the 1984 Food Act. Its findings will be published at a time yet to be determined.'

'The Minister has instructed me to write to you to explain that we cannot at present undertake to respond to letters received from individual members of the public.'

'We have received no complaints about the matter you raise.'

'We are unable at present to allocate any resources to an investigation of the issues you raise.'

'The changes you are suggesting have been tried but met with no success.'

'This is a matter for individual choice and not for government legislation.'

'The products you complain of are sold in large numbers and so clearly fulfil a need.'

'There is no scientific evidence that a significant problem exists.'

Don't be surprised by these sorts of replies. You won't be the first person to be brushed off like this, and you won't be the last. For centuries bureaucracies have fought for the right to protect themselves from interference, and have developed some sophisticated tricks for keeping you confused. If you press for changes they will put up these brick walls, and hope you will go away.

Getting to grips

What is needed to overcome these stubborn but powerful interests? First, we need well-informed consumers, able to see when they are being duped. This book is designed to help consumers become better informed and better able to act.

Second, we need to know who to lobby and who to complain to. We need to know where the power to change things lies, and how to best influence that power in our interests. Again, we have tried to give a little of the insight needed into who controls what in this book.

Third, we need to recruit effective advocates – people who can act on our behalf and stand up for what we want. Consumer organisations set themselves up to perform this role, and we have included a guide to the relevant ones in the address lists.

SUPPORT AND ADVICE

In this section we indicate the people you might turn to when you want to do something about children's food. We list the local authorities who are responsible for social service facilities, for local educational facilities, and who also monitor the quality of the food we are sold, and the labelling and selling of food. We list the health authority staff who can provide support and advice, and who may help you organise meetings and mount exhibitions.

We list some of the many voluntary organisations who can provide information or a local contact. We list the government departments responsible for regulating our food and changing the law. And we list the major baby food companies where you can write when you want to say what you feel about their products.

Local authorities

Local authorities are responsible for, among many other things, the provision of nurseries and the regulation of private under 5s facilities, for schools (except for the ILEA which, while it remains, is responsible for schools in inner London boroughs) and for environmental health and trading standards.

If you have complaints about the activities of food companies, or want to discuss the policies on nursery or school services, then contact your local authority. We cannot give the addresses and phone numbers for each department, but here are the main Town Hall numbers for each authority in Great Britain.

County or borough	Phone number
Avon	0272–290777
Barking & Dagenham	01–592 4500
Barnet	01–202 8282
Barnsley	0226–203232
Bedfordshire	0234–63222
Berkshire	0734–875444
Bexley	01–303 7777
Birmingham	021–235 2037
Bolton	00204–22311
Borders	08352–53301
Brent	01–903 1400
Bromley	01–464 3333
Buckinghamshire	0296–5000
Bury	061–764 6000
Cambridgeshire	0223–317111
Camden	01–278 4444
Central	0786–73111
Cheshire	0244–602424
City of London Corp	01–606 3030

Cleveland	0642–248155
Clwyd	0352–2121
Cornwall	08727–4282
Coventry	0203–25555
Croydon	01–686 4433
Cumbria	0228–23456
Derbyshire	0629–3411
Devon	0392–77977
Doncaster	0302–734444
Dorset	0305–63131
Dudley	0384–55433
Dumfries & Galloway	0387–3141
Durham	0385–64411
Dyfed	0267–233333
Ealing	01–579 2424
East Sussex	0273–475400
Enfield	01–366 6565
Essex	0245–267222
Fife	0592–754411
Gateshead	0632–771011
Gloucestershire	0452–21444
Grampian	0224–682222
Greenwich	01–854 8888
States of Guernsey	0481–27412
Gwent	06333–67711
Gwynedd	0286–4121
Hackney	01–986 3123
Hammersmith & Fulham	01–748 3020
Hampshire	0962–54411
Haringey	01–888 3000
Harrow	01–863 5611
Havering	01–708–46040
Hereford & Worcester	0905–353366
Hertfordshire	0992–54242
Highland	0463–234121
Hillingdon	0895–50111
Hounslow	01–570 7728
Humberside	0482–867131
ILEA	01–633 5000
Isle of Man	0624–26262
Isle of Wight	098352–4031

Islington	01–226 1234
States of Jersey	0534–27286
Kensington & Chelsea	01–937 5464
Kent	0622–671411
Kingston upon Thames	01–546 2121
Knowsley	051–548 6555
Lambeth	01–274 7722
Lancashire	0772–54868
Leicestershire	0533–871313
Lewisham	01–690 4343
Lincolnshire	0522–29931
Liverpool	051–227 3911
Lothian	031–229 9292
Manchester	061–236 3377
Merton	01–946 8070
Mid Glamorgan	0222–28033
Newcastle upon Tyne	0632–328520
Newham	01–472–1430
Norfolk	0603–611122
Northamptonshire	0604–34833
Northumberland	0670–514343
Northern Ireland	0232–647151
North Tyneside	0632–575544
North Yorkshire	0609–3123
Nottinghamshire	0602–823823
Oldham	061–624 0505
Orkney Islands	0856–3535
Oxfordshire	0865–722422
Powys	0597–3711
Redbridge	01–478 3020
Richmond upon Thames	01–891 1411
Rochdale	0706–47474
Rotherham	0709–2121
St Helens	0744–24061
Sandwell	021–569 2200
Sefton	051–992 4040
Sheffield	0742–26444
Shetland Islands	0595–3535
Shropshire	0743–222100
Solihull	021–705 6789
Somerset	0823–73451

South Glamorgan	0222–499022
South Tyneside	0632–554321
Southwark	01–703 6311
Staffordshire	0785–3121
Stockport	061–480 4949
Strathclyde	041–204 2900
Suffolk	0473–55801
Sunderland	0783–76161
Surrey	01–546 1050
Sutton	01–661 5000
Thameside	061–330 8355
Tayside	0382–23281
Tower Hamlets	01–980 4831
Trafford	061–872 2101
Walsall	0922–21244
Waltham Forest	01–527 5544
Wandsworth	01–871 6060
Warwickshire	0926–493431
Western Isles	0851–3773
West Glamorgan	0792–471111
Westminster	01–828 8070
West Sussex	0243–777100
Wigan	0942–44991
Wiltshire	02214–3641
Wirral	051–638 7070
Wolverhampton	0902–27811

If you need advice on nutrition or on your child's health, or you want to arrange a meeting with a speaker, then contact your local health authority. Health visitors are the first point of contact, but you may also want to talk to dietitians in the Dietetics Department, or ask for speakers for your meeting from the Health Education Department and Community Dental Health Department.

Health Authority departments are found through your local hospital or through your local Community Health Council – these should be listed in your phone directory. Otherwise, here are the Regional Health Authorities who should be able to give you the number you want.

Regional Health Authority	*Phone numbers*
East Anglia (For Cambridgeshire, Norfolk, Suffolk)	0223–61212
Mersey (for Cheshire, Merseyside)	051–236 8464
Northern (for Cleveland, Cumbria, Durham, Northumberland, Newcastle, North Tyneside, Gateshead, South Tyneside, Sunderland)	0632–654188
N. Ireland Central Services	0232–224431
North Western (for Lancashire, Wigan, Bolton, Bury, Rochdale, Salford, Manchester, Oldham, Trafford, Stockport, Tameside)	061–236 9465
Oxford (for Berkshire, Buckinghamshire, Northamptonshire, Oxfordshire)	0865–64861
Scottish Common Services	031–552 6255
South Western (for Avon, Cornwall, Devon, Somerset, Gloucestershire)	0272–423271
Thames, North East (for Essex, City, Camden Barking, Enfield, Hackney, Haringey, Havering, Islington, Newham, Redbridge, Tower Hamlets, Waltham Forest)	01–262 8011

Thames, North West   01–262 8011
  (for Bedfordshire,
  Hertfordshire, Barnet,
  Brent, Ealing, Hammersmith
  and Fulham, Harrow,
  Hillingdon, Hounslow,
  Kensington and Chelsea,
  Westminster)

Thames, South East   0424–222555
  (for East Sussex, Kent,
  Bexley, Greenwich,
  Bromley, Lambeth, Lewisham,
  Southwark)

Thames, South West   01–262 8011
  (for Surrey, West Sussex,
  Croydon, Kingston upon Thames,
  Merton, Richmond upon Thames,
  Sutton, Wandsworth)

Trent   0742–306511
  (For Derbyshire,
  Lincolnshire,
  Leicestershire,
  Nottinghamshire,
  Barnsley, Doncaster,
  Sheffield, Rotherham)

Wessex   0962–63511
  (for Dorset, Hampshire,
  Wiltshire, Isle of Wight)

West Midlands   021–454 4828
  (for Hereford and Worcester,
  Shropshire, Staffordshire,
  Warwickshire, Walsall,
  Wolverhampton, Dudley,
  Sandwell, Birmingham,
  Coventry, Solihull)

Yorkshire   0423–65061
  (for Humberside, North
  Yorkshire, Bradford, Leeds,
  Calderdale, Kirklees,
  Wakefield)

Welsh Health Services   0222–499921

Voluntary organisations

Action Against Allergy
43 The Downs
London SW20 8HG
Tel: 01–947 5082

Association of Breastfeeding Mothers
131 Mayow Road
London SE26 4ZH
Tel: 01–778 4769

Asthma Research Council and Asthma Society
300 Upper Street
London N1 2XX
Tel: 01–226 2260

Baby Milk Action Coalition
34 Blinco Grove
Cambridge CB1 4TS
Tel: 0223–210094

Hyperactive Children's Support Group
59 Meadowside
Angmering
Littlehampton
W. Sussex BN16 4BW

La Leche League
Box BM 3424
London WC1 6XX
Tel: 01–883 7801

London Food Commission
88 Old Street
London EC1V 9AR
Tel: 01–253 9513

Maternity Alliance
15 Brittania Street
London WC1
Tel: 01–837 1265

National Childbirth Trust
9 Queensborough Terrace
London W2 3TB
Tel: 01–221 3833

National Eczema Society
Tavistock House North
Tavistock Square
London WC1H 9SR
TelL: 01–388 4097

National Society for Research into Allergy
PO Box 45
Hinckley
Leicestershire LE10 1JY
Tel: 0455–635212

Pre-School Playgroups Association
61 Kings Cross Road
London WC1
Tel: 01–833 0991

The government departments

Your MP*
House of Commons
Westminster
London SW1
Tel: 01–219 3000

* to find out who your MP is, phone the House of Commons
Library
Tel: 01–219 4272

Ministry of Agriculture, Fisheries and Food
Whitehall Place
London SW1A 2HH
Tel: 01–233 3000

Department of Education and Science
Elizabeth House, York Road, London SE1 7PH
Tel: 01–0934 9000

Department of Health and Social Security
Alexander Fleming House, Elephant and Castle
London SE1 6BY
Tel: 01–407 5522

The companies

Boots
1 Thane Road West
Nottingham NG2 3AA
Tel: 0602–501165

Cow & Gate
Cow & Gate House
Manvers Street
Trowbridge
Wilts BA14 8YX
Tel: 02214–68381

Delrosa
Sterling Winthrop
Winthrop House
Friary
Guildford
Surrey
Tel: 0483–505515

Farleys (and Farex)
Crookes Healthcare
PO Box 94
1 Thane Road West
Nottingham NG2 3AA
Tel. 0602–507431

Heinz
H. J. Heinz Co. Ltd
Hayes Park
Hayes
Middlesex UB4 8Al
Tel: 01–573 7757

Milupa
Milupa House
Hercies Road
Hillingdon
Uxbridge
Middlesex UB10 9NA
Tel: 0895–59851

Ribena (and Lucozade)
Beecham Foods
Beecham House
Great West Road
Brentford
Middlesex TW8 9BD
Tel: 01–560 5151

Robinson's
Colman's of Norwich
Carrow
Norwich NR1 2DD
Tel: 0603–660166

Wyeth
Wyeth Laboratories
Huntercombe Lane South
Taplow
Maidenhead
Berks
Tel: 06286–4377

For other food company addresses you can contact your local library (most companies are listed in the Food Trades Dirctory) or else phone the Food and Drink Federation and ask for their information officer. Tel: 01–836 2460.

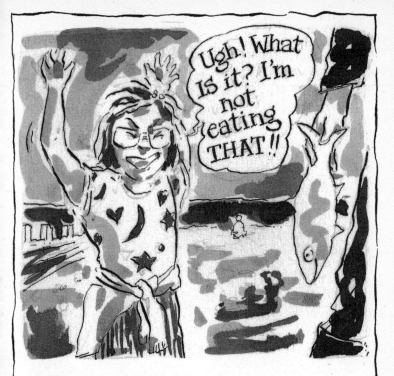

Molly's reached the age of five:
She's shocked to see a fish alive
Without its fingers – O, *great* surprise!
A *head* is there – with mouth – and *eyes!*
O polyphosphate salts, now make
Of minced-up pieces of broken hake
Some fishy digits swelled with water
For Molly's mum to serve her daughter.

7 Getting It Right

GUIDELINES FOR HEALTHY EATING

Despite the feeling that there is conflicting advice on diets, there is actually a remarkable amount of agreement among the more eminent groups of health workers and nutritionists on what is a healthy way of eating for children.

The impression that there is controversy and disagreement is one which benefits the food industry and does no service to anxious parents. Manufacturers of products which are not generally considered important in a healthy diet can always point to 'disagreements among professionals' as a reason for continuing to promote their products. So it should be made clear: in many respects, there is very little disagreement about what is a healthy diet for both adults and children.

The government, the professionals, and consumer organisations have all proposed similar dietary guidelines and similar advice. It should be remembered, though, that the advice is generally made for *groups* of children rather than for single individuals. Individuals, even young children, have their own appetites, their own nutritional needs, their own tastes and preferences, their own growth rates and metabolisms – so that no piece of advice should be applied to a particular child without taking his or her own individual needs and circumstances into account

THE EXPERTS AGREE

The latest document on healthy eating for young children comes from the Department of Health and Social Security, who have recently issued an updated version of their booklet for health professionals giving infant feeding advice, *Present Day Practice in Infant Feeding (1988)*, available from Her Majesty's Stationery Office. It is produced by a group of health professionals (the

Working Party of the Panel on Child Nutrition, of the Committee on Medical Aspects of Food Policy). Although some of the members of this panel are reputed to have rather close relations with commercial food interests, we are assured that they endeavour to put these to one side when they make their judgements and recommendations.

Prior to this, the British Dietetic Association, the professional organisation for dietitians, issued a report in 1987 on the needs of young children entitled *Children's Diet and Change*. Their recommendations were remarkably similar to those later proposed by the DHSS.

And prior to the report from the BDA, the London Food Commission had produed two documents which contained advice on feeding young children. One of these gave dietary guidelines for nursery and playgroup staff, as part of a booklet on healthy eating and food activities, *Food and Drink for Under Fives*, published in 1985. The other document was prepared by the London Food Commission for the BBC's *Parent Programme* as an advice sheet for people writing in after the broadcast of the programme, in 1986. Once again, the advice to be found in these documents was similar in virtually every respect to the later documents from the BDA and the DHSS.

Here is an overview of all these documents, giving the main points on which they are all agreed.

BASIC PRINCIPLES

- For the first six months, the milk used should be breast-milk or an approved modified infant formula.
- Cereals or thickeners should not be put in feeding bottles
- Full-fat cow's milk can be introduced after 6 months. An approved follow-up milk can be used as an alternative, and breast-feeding or modified infant formula can be used up to at least one year.
- Weaning foods can be introduced after 3 to 6 months, and can include puréed cooked vegetables, fruit, lentils, potatoes and ground cereals such as rice and cornmeal.
- Salt should not be added to a baby's food
- Sugar should not be added to a baby's food
- A well-balanced diet should supply all the vitamins needed, but DHSS drops are usually recommended for all children up to age 2 years, and preferably to age 5 years.

- The main sources of nutrients and energy for a child on a mixed diet should be: milk, lean meat, poultry, fish, eggs, cheese, fruit, vegetables, bread and cereals – preferably of the wholegrain type.
- Adding bran for extra fibre is not recommended.
- Sugary foods and drinks are not recommended.
- Fried foods and high-fat foods such as chips, pastry, fatty meat products and crisps should be limited.
- The reasons for inadequate diets include: long-term food refusal; not having enough money to spend on food; misguided ideas about the amounts and types of food needed; chronic sickness. Such children are 'at risk' and need extra attention to their diets.
- If low-fat diets are to be tried then alternative sources of calories should be provided. Full-fat milk should be used to age 2, then if the overall diet and appetite are good semi-skimmed milk can be offered. Skimmed milk for children under five is not recommended, and 'at risk' children should stay on full-fat milk.
- If milk is not tolerated, then nutritious alternatives need to be tried, such as a modified soya milk.
- Whole foods tend to be bulkier than refined foods, and so snacks may be needed between meals to keep up sufficient calories. Snacks such as milk, fruit, bread and sandwiches are preferable to the sugary and fatty snack foods frequently given.
- Whole nuts should be avoided, as the risk of food inhalation is more common in children under 5. Nut purées and nut butters are a suitable alternative. Care should also be taken with other small pieces of hard food such as raw vegetables which do not dissolve easily.
- Overweight children, and children whose parents are overweight, should be weighed regularly and advice given to the parents on how to provide a diet high in essential nutrients but lower in energy.
- Giving advice on healthy food is not enough. Even if based on cheap grains and pulses the suggestions may be unacceptable. To eliminate the problems of malnutrition in children, particularly those due to poverty, healthy, easily prepared, tasty foods should be available to everyone, whatever their income.

In addition to these guiding principles, the second of the London Food Commission documents outlined ways in which these could be made more practical for parents and others responsible for young children. Adapted from the leaflet prepared for the BBC Parent Programme, the advice is as follows:

DAY-TO-DAY PRACTICE

By about 9 to 12 months, children can cope with most foods eaten by the rest of the family. They will discover puddings, biscuits, cakes and sweets – and the habits of a lifetime will be setting in. These early years are the best opportunity to limit the damage.

TIP   To help survive the sweets and biscuits, try to give healthier food whenever you can.

ENCOURAGE	LIMIT
vegetables (best fresh or frozen)	sweet food
	fatty food
fruit (raw or freshly cooked)	sweet drinks
bread, pitta, chapati	processed
lean meat, fish, poultry	meats, pies
potatoes, pasta, rice,	salty snacks
beans, peas, lentils, dahl,	cakes, biscuits,
breakfast cereals (low or no	jams
sugar),	pastries, packet puddings

If you can, offer the healthier food when the child is most hungry, so what happens at other times is less of a disaster. Eating between meals does no harm if the food is healthy.

TIP Children often want snacks. If possible, have something healthy available.

HEALTHIER SNACK IDEAS

- Sandwiches, or rolls, or pitta, filled with e.g. peanut butter, cottage cheese, banana
- Fruit: apples, bananas, satsumas, pears
- Home-made popcorn (no salt or sugar needed)
- Milk or pure fruit juices (best diluted with water)

When it comes to cooking there are several methods which can help to improve the healthiness of the food.

TIP   Here are some tips for more nutritious cooking:

LIMIT	TRY
frying or deep-frying, roasting in fat added salt, fat or skin on meat, hard fats, coconut oil, palm oil, butter or ghee white flour, white rice overcooking vegetables or letting them stand around sugar in recipes (try using half the amount)	stir-frying or grilling, baking or steaming, adding herbs or spices skimming fat off stews, gravy oils e.g. sunflower, corn, soya and olive oil wholemeal flour, whole rice raw vegetables or ones cut small and cooked quickly using dried fruit whole or chopped instead of sugar

---

Sometimes it is necessary to cook a meal in a rush, using packet 'convenience' foods. Some of these are better than others, and it may be worth keeping a stock of the better sorts for making a quick, nutritious meal.

TIP   Keep these convenience foods handy:

USEFUL FOR QUICK MAIN MEALS

Frozen: peas, other vegetables, fish, fish fingers, pizzas.

Tins: tomatoes, other vegetables (but drain off the salty, sugary water), tuna fish, sardines and other fish, baked beans and other beans.

Pasta: quick cook varieties are OK, and look for wholemeal and the green, red, and egg types.

AVOID most made up meat products like pies, burgers, sausages and tinned meat – which may have a lot of fat, salt, colourings and preservatives.

Occasionally it can be useful to get a take-away meal. This can be quick and convenient, but may be high in fats and salt.

TIP   If you have the choice, try these:

THE BETTER TAKE-AWAYS

- Pizzas: some chains even do wholemeal pizzas.
- Baked potatoes: choose a low-fat filling.
- Chinese: go for steamed and stir-fried dishes, have lots of rice, avoid fatty meats and rich sauces.
- Indian: as with Chinese, avoid rich dishes and go for vegetable curries, and drier meats like tandoori, and have chapatis, rice, dahl and channa (chickpeas).
- Greek: Doner kebabs are high-fat, but grilled shish kebabs are better – and have pitta, humus and salad.

Battles with children can be at their worst when it comes to sweets and chocolates. If Granny gives Rosie some sweets there is no point snatching the packet away and upsetting them both. A quiet word with Granny might be useful, suggesting healthier foods or toys instead.

TIP   When dentists have children of their own they remember the golden rule: *frequency is worse than quantity*. A small amount of sweetness in the mouth every half-hour is much worse than a big pile of sweets once in the day.

Some dentists have a home rule: 'sweets at meal-times only' or even 'sweets at weekends only'. They make ice-lollies from fruit juice or frozen bananas. And they give their children fluoride supplements if there isn't much fluoride in the water.

These tips apply as much to adults as they do to children. And children need to feel that adults eat the same things they eat – raw carrots or sardines on toast are OK because *you* eat them too. But here are a few words that particularly apply to children between 1 and 5 years old.

- MILK   Whole milk is usually recommended up to 2 years old. Then, if the child is growing well and eats a variety of foods, semi-skimmed milk can be offered. Drinking a lot of milk – say two pints a day – may spoil the appetite for other food.
- NUTS   Pieces of nut do not dissolve easily, and cause problems if caught in the throat or inhaled. It is best to avoid them

until the child is chewing and swallowing well – say by 3 or 4 years old. Nut butters, such as smooth peanut butter, are fine.

- VITAMINS A well-balanced diet should give a child all the vitamins needed. But the DHSS recommends extra vitamins, and these can be obtained very cheaply from the health visitor or local children's clinic.
- ADDITIVES Most additives are used to make food seem more attractive. They are 'cosmetics' for the food – the colours, flavourings, texturisers, flavour enhancers, bulking agents, emulsifiers, and even the preservatives and anti-oxidants which keep the food looking fresh and germ-free when it is months old. So a long list of 'E' numbers might make you suspicious. If you follow the tips given above you will find you are buying less additive-laden food anyway.

Will it work?

Will children actually eat the healthy food, when they know they could always scream for cakes, puddings, sweets? The answer is yes, but it may require some imagination. A lot depends on *presentation*. Look at what food companies do. Ask yourself: what tricks have they used to make their products look attractive to children? Try mixtures of colours, unusual shapes, various textures, attractive wrappings, funny names: 'baby' carrots, 'monster' pie, or themes involving animals, dolls or magic.

Is it expensive? Healthy eating need not cost a lot more – though it depends how much you are spending already. Some nurseries have found that cutting back on processed foods, especially processed meats, and offering healthy snacks, has actually cost less and led to less food being wasted as well. For parents, if money is tight then do make sure you are getting all the welfare benefits and support you are entitled to. Millions of pounds are left unclaimed each year, so check with your local Citizens' Advice Bureau or Welfare Rights Office.

Lastly, if you think that all the tips and advice mean too much change then don't try it all at once. Make changes gradually. If you have any doubts about a child's growth or health, then contact the health visitor, or go to the clinic or visit your doctor. They are there to advise you, so do make use of them.

DO HEALTHY CHILDREN NEED PILLS?

Throughout this book we have been emphasising the trend of the food industry towards providing food with more calories and fewer nutrients than growing children need, even though manufacturers may try to compensate by sprinkling on extra 'powdered vitamin pills' or other supplements.

Anxious parents may even feel they should provide extra insurance by getting their little ones to swallow food supplements, vitamin pills, capsules, lozenges, and all the other paraphernalia that line the shelves of the so-called 'health food' shops. Is this really the answer? It is expensive. It is easy to be muddled by the packets and bottles. And it speaks of the despair of parents who cannot be sure they are getting the right food into their children. They want the best for their children, but is this the best?

We saw in the chapter on weaning foods how the history of the discovery of vitamins shows that we cannot be sure we have got to the end of the list. We cannot know if a bottle of 'multivitamin plus' or 'complete vitamin supplement' really *is* complete, or whether new and important nutrients may still be discovered. The same goes for the minerals – with the further complication that giving too much of one mineral may inhibit the body's ability to get what it needs of another mineral.

A dietitian's response to these confusing problems is to say: eat a well-balanced healthy diet and you will get all you need, in the amounts your body wants and can use. If the body gets these nutrients it will be well nourished, and if it is well nourished it will be better at coping with all the environmental hazards it may have to face – the illnesses, the allergy-causing chemicals, the toxins and the poisons. *If the diet is good, then the only people to benefit from vitamin pills are the people who make and sell them.*

Common or garden nourishment

Children can get the nutrients they need without you having to reach for the pills and supplements. They just need to eat healthily. Eating healthily means having a nutritionally balanced diet. But what is a *healthy balance*? Traditionally this has meant a selection of foods providing plenty of proteins, fats and carbohydrates, which have been considered essential elements for body growth and metabolism.

But in Britain today, the common diseases are related to eating too much of the fats and refined carbohydrates, unnecessary amounts of protein, and not enough of the fibre-rich fruits, vegetables, grains and pulses that our bodies are best adapted to. So the emphasis of *balance* nowadays is towards more fresh and wholesome foods, and away from the rich calorie-dense foods that have become too much a part of our national diet.

What does this mean for planning a weekly menu? It means thinking how you can introduce more vegetables and pulses, and cut back on fatty foods. It means more fruits and less sugary foods. And it means more emphasis on lean cuts of the 'red' meats and on 'white' meats like fish and poultry, and less emphasis on fatty red meats and processed meat products, which tend to be laden with saturated fats.

The recommendation nowadays is to include in a balanced diet something from each of the four groups:

Group 1   Cereal foods and starchy vegetables – wholemeal bread, pasta, rice, potatoes, yams and the like.
Group 2   Fruits and vegetables, especially fresh (if possible) or frozen.
Group 3   Meat and alternatives, including fish and poultry, eggs, nuts, lentils and beans.
Group 4   Milk and milk products, such as yoghurt and cheese.

The emphasis is to provide lots of food from groups 1 and 2, and smaller amounts from groups 3 and 4. In addition, there should be plenty of *water* available to drink.

Small amounts from two groups of refined foods can also be eaten:

Group 5   Sugar, sugary foods and drinks.
Group 6   Butter, margarine, fats and oils.

Foods from these last two groups add energy and, in the case of the fats and oils, some useful polyunsaturated fatty acids. But these foods should not replace food from the four main groups.

Good diets – no problem!

Just to put our minds at rest, in case there are any worries about creating a healthy and balanced diet for a child, we can look a bit more closely at what the foods in the groups above are providing. We can take a shortlist of the main nutrients that we know children need, and ask: what foods, in the groups above, are good sources of these nutrients?

In Table 7.1 there is a listing of the main vitamins and minerals which children need, and the foods that can provide these. Please remember that the figures are *average*. This means the foods will provide these nutrients *on average*, and it means that the recommended amounts of nutrients needed by children are estimated as the *average needed for a group of children*, with some children needing more and some needing less. In many cases these recommended amounts are set at a higher level than actually necessary, just to be safe. The recommended amounts are those given by the Department of Health and Social Security (or the World Health Organisation where indicated). The food nutrient values are from standard food tables (McCance and Widdowson, *The Composition of Foods*, 1985).

Table 7.1 Rich sources of nutrients

Nutrient	Recommended average daily amount	Rich sources
Protein	Under 1: 15–25g 1 to 6: 30–45g 7 to 12: 45–70g	*5g in each of these:* 4oz cooked dahl, beans, peas or rice 1–2 fish or lean meat 1 oz cheddar cheese
Vitamin A (retinol)	Under 1: 450ug 1 to 6: 300ug 7 to 12: 400–750ug	*100ug in each of these:* 1 oz sweet potato, spinach 0.5 oz carrot 1 oz cheese 1 egg yolk 0.5 pint whole milk

Vitamin B1 (thiamine)	Under 1: 0.3mg 1 to 6: 0.5–0.7mg 7 to 12: 0.7–1.0mg	*0.1mg in each of these*: 1 slice wholemeal bread 1 oz lean pork 0.5 oz raw peanuts 0.5 pint milk 1 oz cheddar cheese
Vitamin B2 (riboflavin)	Under 1: 0.4mg 1 to 6: 0.6–0.9mg 7 to 12: 1.0–1.4mg	*0.2mg in each of these*: 2 oz tinned sardines 0.5 pint milk 1 small pot yoghurt 1 egg 4 oz lean meat or chicken 2 oz mushrooms 4 oz broccoli
Vitamin C (ascorbic acid)	Under 1: 20mg 1 to 6: 20mg 7 to 12: 20–25mg	*10mg in each of these*: 3–4 oz potatoes 2 oz cabbage 0.5 oz Brussels sprouts Quarter orange 0.2 oz blackcurrants
Calcium	Under 1: 0.6g 1 to 6: 0.6g 7 to 12: 0.6–0.7g	*0.1g in each of these*: 0.5 oz cheddar cheese 1 oz spinach 1 oz tinned sardines 1 small pot yoghurt Quarter pint milk 2 oz almond or brazil nuts
Iron	Under 1: 6mg 1 to 6: 7–10mg 7 to 12: 10–12mg	*2mg in each of these*: 2 slices wholemeal bread 4 oz lean beef 0.5 oz liver 2 oz tinned sardines 3 oz cooked beans, lentils 2 oz spinach
Zinc*	Under 1: 3–5mg 1 to 6: 10mg 7 to 12: 10–15mg	*2mg in each of these*: 2–3 slices wholemeal bread 2 oz lean beef, lamb 1 oz liver 2 oz peanuts, other nuts

*WHO Guidelines.
Source   LFC; DHSS RDAs; McCance and Widdowson.

YOU KNOW BEST

There is one way a parent or relative or guardian knows whether their child is doing well or not: by looking carefully. Usually the signs are there – a tired sickly child, a child with no appetite, a child that isn't growing well . . . and that is where an *early warning* can be useful.

For several years health workers in underdeveloped countries have been keeping an eye on the health of young children by watching their progress on a *Road to Health* chart. This is a simplified form of weight chart of the sort used by paediatricians to plot the weights of babies and see how they are progressing. Gradually these are being recognised as a valuable educational tool for mothers to monitor their children, too, and see when the weights start showing a trend away from the normal growth patterns.

A *Road to Health chart* (Figs. 7.1–7.2) is easy to use: all you have to know is your child's weight and age. Whenever you wish, preferably at regular intervals (e.g. monthly) you mark the child's weight on the graph, above the child's age at that time. Then join that mark to the previous mark to get a continuous line from the starting date to the present date.

Here is an example:

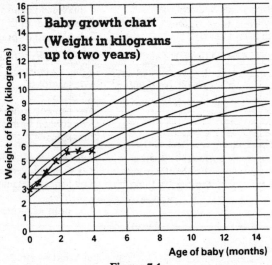

Figure 7.1

The latest weight is about 5.5 kg (or 5,500 grams). This is marked above the child's present age, and by joining this point to the previous point we can see a trend developing. The trend in this case is *away* from the average middle of the road band, and is heading towards the 'bottom 5 per cent' line. This indicates an early warning of something beginning to go wrong. The child has not actually lost weight, and is not yet seriously underweight, but the *trend* suggests that things may get worse in the next few weeks. It is spotting the trend developing that gives an early warning, and so indicates that it is time to take the child to the clinic, remembering to take the baby's chart along to show what it is that makes you concerned. It may be nothing, or it may be something which can easily be put right at this early stage.

Most babies will show weight gains along the middle of the road band, and some will travel along the two bands either side of the middle. A few will continue along the outside. What matters most is a change away from the middle towards the sides of the road or off the sides completely. If you see this change developing then get advice from a midwife, health visitor or doctor.

Here is a blank chart for children aged nought to two.

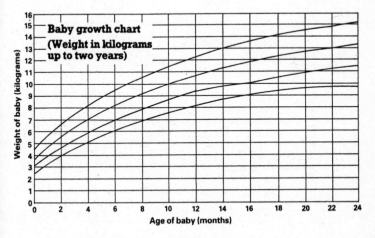

Figure 7.2

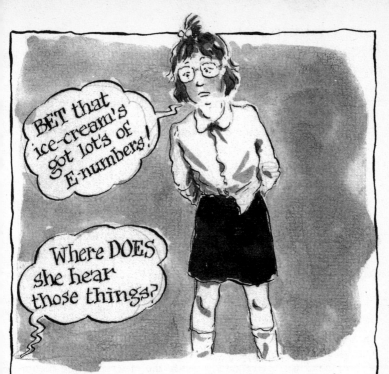

O processor, relax. Now Moll is six!
Though playgroup taught the girl
                              some tricks
(Her teachers, spurning packet goods
Gave Moll a taste for fresh-made foods,
Vegetables—hand-cut by kids—and pasta,
Beans and pulses) 'twas no disaster.
Moll's now at school; lax laws are handy
For selling crisps, coke, pies and candy.

A CHARTER FOR CHILDREN'S FOOD

Here are some examples of the practical changes that can be campaigned for, and which would form the beginning of a movement towards better food for our children:

Clear Standards

1　The present Recommended Daily Allowances for nutrients need to be expanded, and an indication of maximum and minimum allowances specified. Safe and adequate levels of all nutrients for children should be established, which cover the full spectrum of nutrients, and against which average diets in Britain can be evaluated.

Careful Monitoring

2　The food eaten by children at present should be regularly monitored on a large scale, as should those aspects of children's health and development where nutrition is thought to play a role. These need to be evaluated against the criteria of the recommended safe and adequate levels. The needs of vulnerable groups in the population need to be looked at with particular emphasis.

Agreed Goals

3　In the light of the monitoring of children's diets suggested in (2) above, medium- and long-term goals need to be set that will ensure that the diets meet the standards set in (1) above.

School Meals Standards

4　Nutritional standards for school meals need to be reintroduced. These were abandoned in 1980 with further lowering of quality when school meals were not required to be provided except to those on welfare benefits. School dinners, and other food provided to young children in large-scale facilities, provide an excellent opportunity for establishing healthy diets, and for demonstrating to parents the 'authoritative' standards which can be achieved.

Unnecessary Additives Restricted

5   Non-nutritive additives in children's food which cannot be justified strictly on health grounds need to be severely restricted. One might say this should apply to adults too, but for children, especially young children, the element of informed choice is missing: they don't know and might not understand what effects the not-strictly-necessary additives may have on their health and should not be asked to make choices. Healthy food can be and needs to be attractive without resorting to added cosmetics.

Preventive Health on the Syllabus

6   As part of their regular school syllabus, children need to be taught the essentials of good nutrition and the reality of food provision in Britain. The sources of our food, farming techniques and medical effects of our diets need to be covered. Material provided by the food industry to schools should be rejected, or used for teaching only as a means of showing its partisan nature.

Consumer Research Priorities

7   Government research priorities need to be removed from the hands of the food industry. Food research needs to be funded by impartial research centres, which do not rely on food industry money, and which have their priorities set by committees on which consumer representatives are in the majority, or even form the entire membership.

No Secrets
8   Government advisory committees need to be fully open to public view. The proceedings of these committees would be open to public scrutiny, the reports would be entirely public, and the role of interested parties confined to presenting their evidence and stating their cases. They would not be able to vote.

Independent Data Sources

9   Consumers need continuous and reliable sources of information. Consumer groups need to be supported in their work without having to rely on charitable donations or private spon-

sorship. Opportunities for national discussion and the expression of consumer concerns need to be created to ensure that such groups represent their client interests.

Vested Interests Declared

10   Any politician being paid by or having financial interests in food should make these clear whenever they make statements on food policies, and their voting on these matters should be restricted.

Labelling Laws Tightened

11   Food should be labelled in the same way that clothing is labelled – with a list of the quantities of each ingredient. Labelling should also be more explicit – for example, saying which species of animal, and what parts of an animal's body, are being used in meat products. Nutritional labelling should include the current concerns of salt and added salt, sugar and added sugar (in all forms), various fats and added fats, and also indicate (as it does in the United States) what levels of vitamins and minerals can be expected.

Food Inspectors' Powers Strengthened

12   Increased resources and increased powers need to be made available to the food inspectors and enforcement departments, who have the responsibility for monitoring the quality of our food. Public analysts, trading standards officers and environmental health inspectors need greater support in their work, and better means of communicating the results of their work to the public.

Highest EEC Standards

13   The present approach to the 'unified market' of the EEC needs to be reconsidered as it may lower overall food standards. Instead, standards need to be adopted in Britain which reflect the highest prevailing in Europe: if one country bans a colouring agent then we will too, if another forbids pork fat added to beefburgers then we will too.

Environment Conserved

14   Food policies should conserve our natural resources and protect our environment for future generations. No food, food-additive or food-related technology which is banned in Britain should be exported to other countries.

These proposals form the basis for a children's food charter, to ensure that future generations benefit from the lessons we have had to learn.

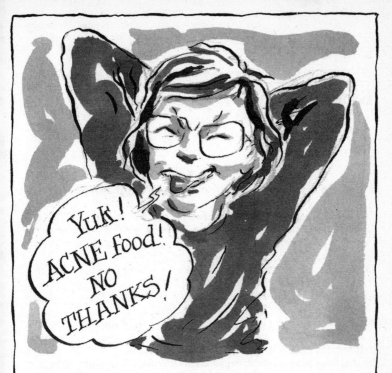

But what is this? The Kids close ranks—
"Yuk! Acne food!" cries Moll "No thanks!
"I'll take packed lunch to school instead!"
"You won't" says Mum, and sees the Head
To ask for salads, jacket spuds,
Wholemeal bread, low sugar puds.
Yet all's not lost: Moll's greatest treat
Remains Mechanically Recovered Meat.

Bibliography

Peggy Brusseau, *Let's Cook It Together* (Wellingborough: Thorson, 1986).

Geoffrey Cannon, *The Politics of Food* (London: Century, 1987).

Isobel Cole-Hamilton and Tim Lang, *Tightening Belts: A Report on the Impact of Poverty on Food* (London: London Food Commission, 1986).

Department of Health and Social Security, *Prevention and Health – Eating for Health* (London: HMSO, 1978).

Department of Health and Social Security, *Present Day Practice in Infant Feeding*, 1988 edn (London: HMSO, 1988).

Mary Goodwin and Gerry Pollen, *Creative Food Experiences for Children*, revised edn (Washington, DC: Center for Science in the Public Interest, 1980).

Health Education Council, *Proposals for Nutrition Guidelines for Health Education in Britain* (The NACNE Report) (London: HEC, 1983).

Roberta Bishop Johnson, *Wholefood for the Whole Family* (Illinois: La Leche League International, 1981).

Felicity Lawrence (ed)., *Additives: Your Complete Survival Guide* (London: Century, 1986).

Tim Lobstein, *Food and Drink for Under Fives* (London: London Food Commission, 1985).

Maureen Minchin, *Breastfeeding Matters* (London: Alma Publications and George Allen & Unwin: Sydney, 1985).

McCance and Widdowson, Food Composition Tables, 4th edition, edited by A. A. Paul and D. A. Southgate (London: HMSO, 1977).

Caroline Walker and Geoffrey Cannon, *The Food Scandal* (London: Century, 1984).

Jan Walsh, *The Meat Machine* (London: Columbus Books, 1986).

Gillian Weaver, *Feeding Time: How to Cope with Your Child's Eating Problems* (London: Columbus Books, 1985).

World Health Organisation, *International Code of Marketing of Breastmilk Substitutes* (Geneva: WHO, 1981).

John Yudkin, *Pure White and Deadly*, 2nd edn (Harmondsworth: Penguin Books, 1988).

Index

THE LONDON FOOD COMMISSION

FOOD ADULTERATION

'ALL NATURAL: NO ARTIFICIAL COLOURS OR FLAVOURS'

This is an increasingly familiar claim made for the food we buy. But what about the other ingredients? Additives are only one form of adulteration. Nitrates, excess water, pesticide residues, too much fat, and newest of them all food irradiation, are some of the others. The questions they pose for all of us are inescapable, as is the overall issue of poor quality food dressed up to be what it is not.

In this book the London Food Commission, Britain's independent food watchdog, spells out the dangers, and suggests solutions. It challenges official policy and condemns official secrecy. It says why British food is the sick food of Europe. It believes that what is needed is a major shake-up in Whitehall and the food trades, and calls for a new anti-adulteration alliance — a positive campaign for improved food policy. And it backs all its arguments with rigorous and detailed evidence.

Food matters to everyone. We deserve the best. We will only get it if we demand it. This book spells out what our demands should be.